3D Innovations in Personalized Surgery

3D Innovations in Personalized Surgery

Editors

Joep Kraeima
Sebastiaan de Visscher
Max Witjes

MDPI • Basel • Beijing • Wuhan • Barcelona • Belgrade • Manchester • Tokyo • Cluj • Tianjin

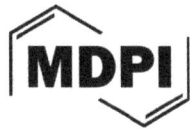

Editors

Joep Kraeima
3D LAB and OMFS
Groningen
Groningen
Netherlands

Sebastiaan de Visscher
OMFS
Groningen
Groningen
Netherlands

Max Witjes
3D Lab and OMFS
Groningen
Groningen
Netherlands

Editorial Office
MDPI
St. Alban-Anlage 66
4052 Basel, Switzerland

This is a reprint of articles from the Special Issue published online in the open access journal *Journal of Personalized Medicine* (ISSN 2075-4426) (available at: www.mdpi.com/journal/jpm/special_issues/3D_Personalized_Surgery).

For citation purposes, cite each article independently as indicated on the article page online and as indicated below:

LastName, A.A.; LastName, B.B.; LastName, C.C. Article Title. *Journal Name* **Year**, *Volume Number*, Page Range.

ISBN 978-3-0365-6484-5 (Hbk)
ISBN 978-3-0365-6483-8 (PDF)

© 2023 by the authors. Articles in this book are Open Access and distributed under the Creative Commons Attribution (CC BY) license, which allows users to download, copy and build upon published articles, as long as the author and publisher are properly credited, which ensures maximum dissemination and a wider impact of our publications.
The book as a whole is distributed by MDPI under the terms and conditions of the Creative Commons license CC BY-NC-ND.

Contents

Joep Kraeima, Sebastiaan de Visscher and Max Witjes
Three-Dimensional Innovations in Personalized Surgery
Reprinted from: *J. Pers. Med.* **2023**, *13*, 113, doi:10.3390/jpm13010113 1

Sherif Idris, Heather Logan, Paul Tabet, Martin Osswald, Suresh Nayar and Hadi Seikaly
The Accuracy of 3D Surgical Design and Simulation in Prefabricated Fibula Free Flaps for Jaw Reconstruction
Reprinted from: *J. Pers. Med.* **2022**, *12*, 1766, doi:10.3390/jpm12111766 3

Nick Assink, Anne M. L. Meesters, Kaj ten Duis, Jorrit S. Harbers, Frank F. A. IJpma and Hugo C. van der Veen et al.
A Two-Step Approach for 3D-Guided Patient-Specific Corrective Limb Osteotomies
Reprinted from: *J. Pers. Med.* **2022**, *12*, 1458, doi:10.3390/jpm12091458 11

Anne M. L. Meesters, Miriam G. E. Oldhoff, Neeltje M. Trouwborst, Nick Assink, Joep Kraeima and Max J. H. Witjes et al.
Quantitative Three-Dimensional Measurements of Acetabular Fracture Displacement Could Be Predictive for Native Hip Survivorship [†]
Reprinted from: *J. Pers. Med.* **2022**, *12*, 1464, doi:10.3390/jpm12091464 21

Bram B. J. Merema, Max J. H. Witjes, Nicolaas B. Van Bakelen, Joep Kraeima and Frederik K. L. Spijkervet
Four-Dimensional Determination of the Patient-Specific Centre of Rotation for Total Temporomandibular Joint Replacements: Following the Groningen Principle
Reprinted from: *J. Pers. Med.* **2022**, *12*, 1439, doi:10.3390/jpm12091439 33

Juliana F. Sabelis, Ruud Schreurs, Harald Essig, Alfred G. Becking and Leander Dubois
Personalized Medicine Workflow in Post-Traumatic Orbital Reconstruction
Reprinted from: *J. Pers. Med.* **2022**, *12*, 1366, doi:10.3390/jpm12091366 47

Bram B. J. Merema, Jelbrich J. Sieswerda, Frederik K. L. Spijkervet, Joep Kraeima and Max J. H. Witjes
A Contemporary Approach to Non-Invasive 3D Determination of Individual Masticatory Muscle Forces: A Proof of Concept
Reprinted from: *J. Pers. Med.* **2022**, *12*, 1273, doi:10.3390/jpm12081273 63

Enkh-Orchlon Batbayar, Nick Assink, Joep Kraeima, Anne M. L. Meesters, Ruud R. M. Bos and Arjan Vissink et al.
Quantitative Three-Dimensional Computed Tomography Measurements Provide a Precise Diagnosis of Fractures of the Mandibular Condylar Process
Reprinted from: *J. Pers. Med.* **2022**, *12*, 1225, doi:10.3390/jpm12081225 77

Nicolaas B. van Bakelen, Jasper W. van der Graaf, Joep Kraeima and Frederik K. L. Spijkervet
Reproducibility of 2D and 3D Ramus Height Measurements in Facial Asymmetry
Reprinted from: *J. Pers. Med.* **2022**, *12*, 1181, doi:10.3390/jpm12071181 89

Peter A. J. Pijpker, Jos M. A. Kuijlen, Katalin Tamási, D. L. Marinus Oterdoom, Rob A. Vergeer and Gijs Rijtema et al.
The Accuracy of Patient-Specific Spinal Drill Guides Is Non-Inferior to Computer-Assisted Surgery: The Results of a Split-Spine Randomized Controlled Trial
Reprinted from: *J. Pers. Med.* **2022**, *12*, 1084, doi:10.3390/jpm12071084 101

Seung-Han Shin, Moo-Sub Kim, Do-Kun Yoon, Jae-Jin Lee and Yang-Guk Chung
Does a Customized 3D Printing Plate Based on Virtual Reduction Facilitate the Restoration of Original Anatomy in Fractures?
Reprinted from: *J. Pers. Med.* **2022**, *12*, 927, doi:10.3390/jpm12060927 . . . . **113**

Haye H. Glas, Joep Kraeima, Silke Tribius, Frank K. J. Leusink, Carsten Rendenbach and Max Heiland et al.
Three-Dimensional Evaluation of Isodose Radiation Volumes in Cases of Severe Mandibular Osteoradionecrosis for the Prediction of Recurrence after Segmental Resection
Reprinted from: *J. Pers. Med.* **2022**, *12*, 834, doi:10.3390/jpm12050834 . . . . **123**

Nathalie Vosselman, Haye H. Glas, Bram J. Merema, Joep Kraeima, Harry Reintsema and Gerry M. Raghoebar et al.
Three-Dimensional Guided Zygomatic Implant Placement after Maxillectomy
Reprinted from: *J. Pers. Med.* **2022**, *12*, 588, doi:10.3390/jpm12040588 . . . . **135**

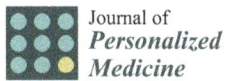

Journal of Personalized Medicine

Editorial

Three-Dimensional Innovations in Personalized Surgery

Joep Kraeima [1,2,*], Sebastiaan de Visscher [1] and Max Witjes [1,2]

1. Department of Oral and Maxillofacial Surgery, University of Groningen, University Medical Center Groningen, 9713 GZ Groningen, The Netherlands
2. 3D Lab, University Medical Center Groningen, University of Groningen, 9713 GZ Groningen, The Netherlands
* Correspondence: j.kraeima@umcg.nl

Citation: Kraeima, J.; de Visscher, S.; Witjes, M. Three-Dimensional Innovations in Personalized Surgery. *J. Pers. Med.* **2023**, *13*, 113. https://doi.org/10.3390/jpm13010113

Received: 22 November 2022
Accepted: 30 November 2022
Published: 4 January 2023

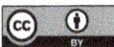

Copyright: © 2023 by the authors. Licensee MDPI, Basel, Switzerland. This article is an open access article distributed under the terms and conditions of the Creative Commons Attribution (CC BY) license (https://creativecommons.org/licenses/by/4.0/).

Due to the introduction of three-dimensional (3D) technology in surgery, it has become possible to preoperatively plan complex bone resections and reconstructions, (corrections and adjustments related to bones), from head to toe. Three-dimensional technology has proven to be a valuable tool for the surgeon, especially when executing complex surgery in the operating room, as crucial decision making with regard to resection margins, planning of osteotomies, screw, and dental implant location is predetermined by virtual planning [1].

Dedicated 3D virtual surgical planning (VSP) software gives a detailed 3D virtual model of the patient based on CT and MRI scans or other imaging modalities, in order to measure, evaluate, simulate or correct parameters that are relevant to the treatment.

This 3D VSP workflow has evolved from a supporting visualization and virtual measurement and evaluation tool to an integrated method that allows for complete pre-operative surgical decision making and designing patient specific implants (designed for surgical procedures) [2].

The use of 3D virtual planning, 3D printing of surgical aids (and parts), as well as navigational technology, is associated with the adage 'plan your operation and operate your plan' [1,3]. The increasing availability and useability of the 3D software and translation instruments, such as 3D-printed guides, has led to the widespread use of some form of 3D technology in healthcare. This has led to improvements in terms of accuracy, predictability and safety for both the surgeon and the patient.

The Next Step

The workflow of 3D VSP and subsequent design of patient-specific implants (PSI) have evolved in recent years as a result of automation and developments in printing.

Automation of the 3D VSP steps can be achieved (as reported in the literature) by means of new segmentation software tools, artificial intelligence applications and other application-specific optimization methods. This leads to faster and less user-dependent preparation of a 3D VSP [4].

Recent developments in the field of 3D printing allow us to develop more complex designs of patient-specific implants, use different materials (for the implants) and optimize the implants' surface. Application of biomechanical models and finite element methods can predict the behavior of, e.g., osteosynthesis plates or implants in a patient, and therefore can be used to improve the design of osteosynthesis materials and implants. In search of further optimization of the design of 3D VSP-based osteosynthesis materials and implants, the output of a FE model should be applied in the design process by means of a topology optimization (TO) process.

This Special Issue, entitled '3D innovations in personalized surgery', presents a series of highly innovative studies and reviews on bone-related applications of the latest 3D technology. These applications include optimization of the 3D VSP, developments in patient-specific biomechanical modeling, inclusion of motion (4D), implant optimizations, surgical navigation and post-operative evaluation of accuracy.

Three-dimensional technology has become the standard-of-care and is expected to bring many more advantages for both the surgeon and the patient in the near future.

Author Contributions: All authors have contributed to the writing and reviewing. All authors have read and agreed to the published version of the manuscript.

Conflicts of Interest: The authors declare no conflict of interest.

References

1. Witjes, M.J.H.; Schepers, R.H.; Kraeima, J. Impact of 3D virtual planning on reconstruction of mandibular and maxillary surgical defects in head and neck oncology. *Curr. Opin. Otolaryngol. Head Neck Surg.* **2018**, *26*, 108–114. [CrossRef] [PubMed]
2. Kraeima, J. *Three Dimensional Virtual Surgical Planning for Patient Specific Osteosynthesis and Devices in Oral and Maxillofacial Surgery. A New Era*; Rijksuniversiteit Groningen: Groningen, Netherlands, 2007; Volume 3, pp. 154–196.
3. Schelkun, S.R. Lessons from aviation safety: "plan your operation—And operate your plan!". *Patient Saf. Surg.* **2014**, *8*, 154–196. [CrossRef] [PubMed]
4. Qiu, B.; van der Wel, H.; Kraeima, J.; Glas, H.H.; Guo, J.; Borra, R.J.H.; Witjes, M.J.H.; van Ooijen, P.M.A. Automatic Segmentation of Mandible from Conventional Methods to Deep Learning—A Review. *J. Pers. Med.* **2021**, *11*, 629. [CrossRef] [PubMed]

Disclaimer/Publisher's Note: The statements, opinions and data contained in all publications are solely those of the individual author(s) and contributor(s) and not of MDPI and/or the editor(s). MDPI and/or the editor(s) disclaim responsibility for any injury to people or property resulting from any ideas, methods, instructions or products referred to in the content.

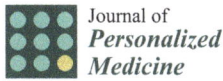

Article

The Accuracy of 3D Surgical Design and Simulation in Prefabricated Fibula Free Flaps for Jaw Reconstruction

Sherif Idris [1], Heather Logan [2], Paul Tabet [1,3], Martin Osswald [1,2], Suresh Nayar [1,2] and Hadi Seikaly [1,2,*]

1. Division of Otolaryngology—Head and Neck Surgery, Department of Surgery, University of Alberta, Edmonton, AB T6G 2B7, Canada
2. Institute for Reconstructive Sciences in Medicine, Misericordia Community Hospital, Edmonton, AB T5R 4H5, Canada
3. Division of Otolaryngology-Head & Neck Surgery, Department of Surgery, Université de Montréal, Montreal, PQ H1T 2M4, Canada
* Correspondence: hseikaly@ualberta.ca; Tel.: +1-(780)-407-3691

Abstract: The ideal jaw reconstruction involves the restoration and maintenance of jaw continuity, jaw relations, joint alignment, and facial contour, and, most importantly, dental occlusal reconstruction. One of the essential requirements of achieving a consistent functional outcome is to place the bony reconstruction in the correct three-dimensional position as it relates to the other jaw segments and dentition. A protocol of occlusion-driven reconstruction of prefabricated fibular free flaps that are customized to the patient with surgical design and simulation (SDS)-planned osseointegrated implant installation was developed by our institution. This innovation introduced significant flexibility and efficiency to jaw reconstructions, but functional and cosmetic outcomes were dependent on the accuracy of the final reconstructions when compared to the SDS plan. The purpose of this study was to examine the accuracy of the SDS-planned fibular flap prefabrication in a cohort of patients undergoing jaw reconstruction. All patients that had undergone primary jaw reconstruction with prefabricated fibular free flaps were reviewed. The primary outcome of this study was the accuracy of the postoperative implant positions as compared to the SDS plan. A total of 23 implants were included in the analysis. All flaps survived, there was no implant loss postoperatively, and all the patients underwent all stages of the reconstruction. SDS planning of fibular flap prefabrication resulted in better than 2 mm accuracy of osteointegrated implant placement in a cohort of patients undergoing jaw reconstruction. This accuracy could potentially result in improved functional and cosmetic outcomes.

Keywords: personalized medicine; dental osseointegrated implants; prefabricated fibula free flap; mandible and maxilla surgery; surgical design and simulation; virtual planning; additive manufacturing

Citation: Idris, S.; Logan, H.; Tabet, P.; Osswald, M.; Nayar, S.; Seikaly, H. The Accuracy of 3D Surgical Design and Simulation in Prefabricated Fibula Free Flaps for Jaw Reconstruction. *J. Pers. Med.* **2022**, *12*, 1766. https://doi.org/10.3390/jpm12111766

Academic Editors: Joep Kraeima, Sebastiaan de Visscher and Max J. H. Witjes

Received: 30 August 2022
Accepted: 30 September 2022
Published: 26 October 2022

Publisher's Note: MDPI stays neutral with regard to jurisdictional claims in published maps and institutional affiliations.

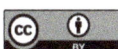

Copyright: © 2022 by the authors. Licensee MDPI, Basel, Switzerland. This article is an open access article distributed under the terms and conditions of the Creative Commons Attribution (CC BY) license (https://creativecommons.org/licenses/by/4.0/).

1. Introduction

The ideal jaw reconstruction involves the restoration and maintenance of jaw continuity, jaw relations, joint alignment, and facial contour, and, most importantly, dental occlusal reconstruction. One of the essential requirements of achieving a consistent functional outcome is to place the bony reconstruction in the correct three-dimensional (3D) position as it relates to the other jaw segments and dentition. This occlusion-driven reconstruction of the jaws was first described in 2003 by Rohner et al. [1].

The use of surgical design and simulation (SDS) in head and neck reconstruction has increased over the past decade. Surgery is planned virtually and, once completed, the SDS-planned reconstruction is translated back to a physical plan that can be implemented in the operating room using various tools and guides. Studies have demonstrated that SDS can reduce surgical time, ischemia time, and inaccuracies compared to analog planning [1–8]. SDS-assisted reconstructions maintain 3D spatial relationships of the reconstruction and are essential when reestablishing dental occlusion with osseointegrated implants [9–11].

An occlusion-driven reconstruction protocol of prefabricated fibular free flaps with SDS-planned osseointegrated implant installation was developed by the Division of Otolaryngology—Head and Neck Surgery at the University of Alberta and the Institute of Reconstructive Sciences in Medicine in Edmonton, AB, Canada [12]. This innovation introduced significant flexibility and efficiency to reconstructions. We also developed surgical tools which, in combination with a set of instruments and components (FIRST System, Southern Implants, Irene, South Africa), allowed the transfer of the SDS plan as a custom, fully guided resection and reconstruction procedure for the patient in the operating room.

The accuracy of the final reconstructions when compared to the SDS plan is essential for achieving a functional occlusion and cosmetic outcomes [12]. The purpose of this study was to examine the accuracy of the SDS modifications of fibular flap prefabrication in a cohort of patients undergoing jaw reconstruction.

2. Material and Methods

2.1. Study Design

The University of Alberta Health Research Ethics Board approved this study on 26 November 2019. (Pro00096288). The cohort of patients were followed prospectively.

2.2. Patients

All patients that had undergone primary jaw reconstruction with prefabricated fibular free flaps were reviewed. Six had completed their treatment protocol and were included in the final analysis.

2.3. Virtual Surgical Planning

Each patient had a high-resolution helical Computed Tomography (CT) scan of the facial bones and the fibula. Images were stored in an uncompressed Digital Communications in Medicine (DICOM) format. These files were imported into Mimics Medical 17.0 software (Materialise, Leuven, Belgium) and were then segmented and reconstructed into 3D digital models.

The virtual surgical planning was carried out using Geomagic Freeform software (3D Systems, SC, USA) during a web-based online planning session between the primary reconstructive head and neck surgeon, a maxillofacial prosthodontist, and a surgical simulationalist at the Medical Modeling Research Laboratory at the Institute for Reconstructive Sciences in Medicine, Misericordia Community Hospital, Edmonton, AB, Canada. During this planning session, the resection planes of the jaw were established based on the surgeon's clinical judgment. Participants in the planning session were able to simultaneously view 3D representations of the patients' anatomy, plan optimal implant positions based on the patients' native dentition, perform virtual resections of the jaws, and plan the fibular reconstruction position based on the planned implant positions (Figure 1).

Using the virtual surgical plan, a patient-specific fibular implant guide was fabricated for the Stage I surgery, and additional patient-specific surgical guides were fabricated for the Stage II surgery. Specifically, a fibula osteotomy guide, patient-specific reference models of the fibula, presurgical models, planned reconstruction models, and mandible or maxillofacial resection cutting guides, were created for Stage II. All models were manufactured using 3D printers and sterilized for surgical use.

2.4. Surgical Procedure

2.4.1. Stage I: Flap Prefabrication

The surgical implant drilling guide was mounted on the fibula in the predetermined position, and the osseointegrated dental implants were instilled. Next, an impression (with dental impression materials) of the final positions of the implants was taken to aid in the design of future dental prostheses. The fibula and implants were then covered with a split-thickness skin graft and a Gore-Tex® patch (Preclude® Dura Substitute, W.L. Gore & Associates, Inc., Flagstaff, AZ, USA) as described by Rohner et al. [1] (Figure 2).

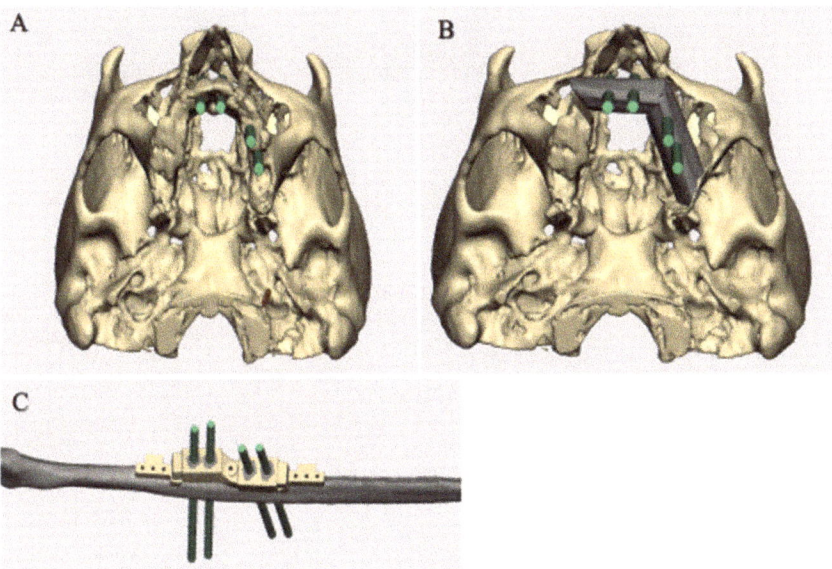

Figure 1. SDS planning. (**A**) Optimal implant positions based on the patient's native dentition were confirmed. (**B**) The resection planes of the jaw were established. (**C**) The position of the fibula reconstruction based on the planned implant positions.

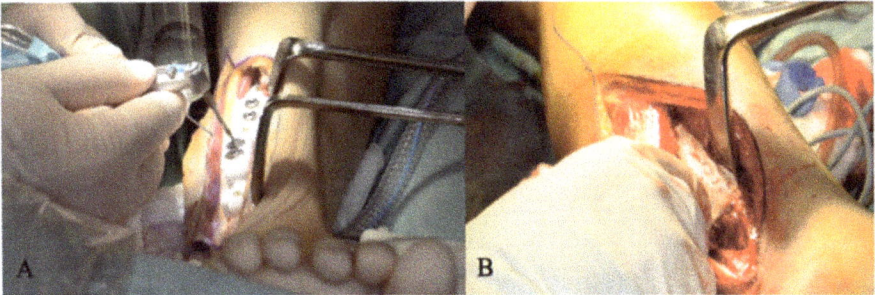

Figure 2. (**A**) Three-dimension printed drilling guide is anchored to the fibula and osseointegrated implants are placed in the planned location. (**B**) Split-thickness skin graft placed over the lateral aspect of the fibula containing the implants.

2.4.2. Stage II: Jaw Reconstruction

Six months after Stage I, the jaw resection and fibula reconstruction were performed. The fibula was re-exposed and removal of the Gore-Tex® membrane revealed the newly attached epithelial tissue around the implants and along the lateral sides of the fibula (Figure 3A). The flap was elevated and placed into a fibular holder (Southern Implants, Irene, South Africa) to maintain vascularization and safe manipulation of the flap during surgery (Figure 3B). The surgical cutting guide was repositioned on the implants, and the fibula was further osteotomized as indicated by the patient-specific fibular cutting guide produced by SDS based on the preoperative virtual surgical plan (Figure 3C). Proper configuration of the bone segments according to the planned digital design was achieved by mounting the interim dental prosthesis on the osseointegrated implants (Figure 3D)

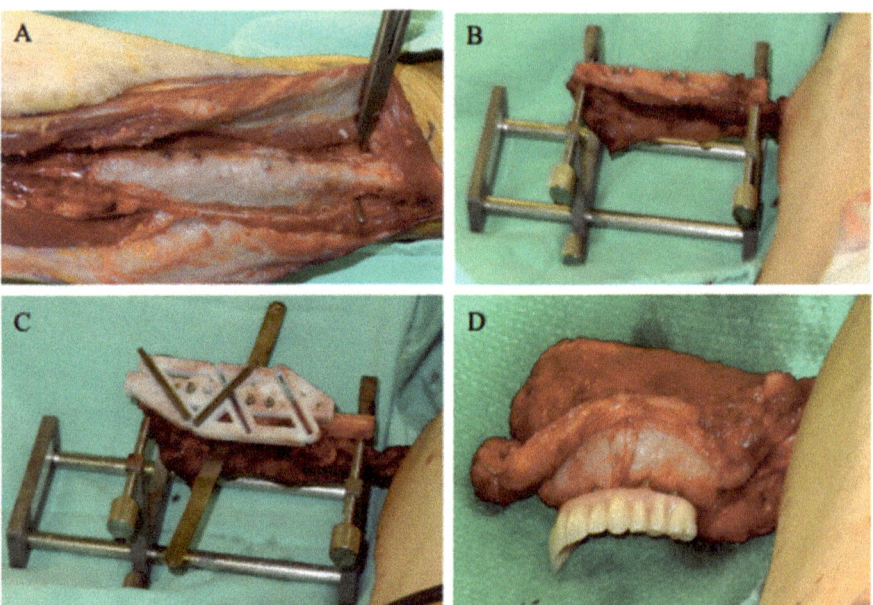

Figure 3. (**A**) Fibula was re-exposed, and removal of the Gore-Tex® membrane revealed the newly attached epithelial tissue around the implants and along the lateral sides of the fibula. (**B**) The flap was placed into a fibular holder (Southern Implants, Irene, South Africa) so that the flap could be safely manipulated during surgery while remaining vascularized. (**C**) The surgical cutting guide was repositioned on the implants, and the fibula was further osteotomized. (**D**) Proper configuration of the bone segments was established, with the interim dental prosthesis on the osseointegrated implants. The construct was relocated to the jaw and the flap was plated to the jaw using mini plates.

The flap and transfer template construct were relocated to the jaw, and the patient was placed in occlusion, with the construct in the accurate spatial relationship. The bone segment(s) of the flap were plated to the jaw using mini plates. Finally, soft tissue adjustment and microvascular anastomoses were performed.

2.4.3. Stage III: Prosthodontic Treatment

The definitive dental prosthesis was fabricated and delivered after healing was complete (Figure 4).

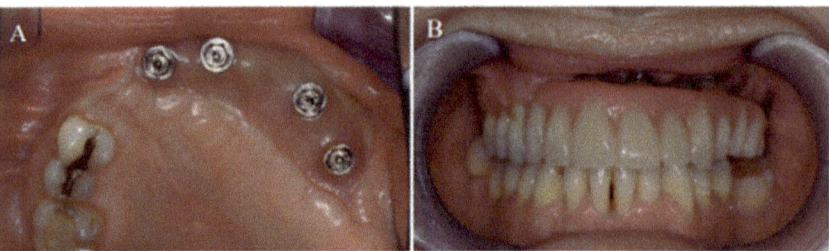

Figure 4. (**A**) Complete osseointegration of the dental implants into the neomandible. (**B**) Placement of the final acrylic dental prosthesis).

2.5. Primary Outcome

The primary outcome of this study was the accuracy of the postoperative implant positions as compared to the SDS plan. Each patient had a high-resolution helical CT scan of the facial bones using either a Somatom Sensation (Siemens, Germany) or a GE VCT (GE Healthcare, Waukesha, WI) 64-slice CT select scanner via a 0.625 mm collimation with a 25.0 cm field of view and 0 degree gantry tilt. All patients had postoperative CT scans of their facial bones 6–12 months after the Stage II procedure.

2.6. Data Analysis

The preoperative digital plan, referred to as "planned", and the scans of the postoperative results, referred to as "actual", were used for our analysis. Digitally placed spheres (1 mm diameter) were manually positioned in the geometric center of the planned and actual implant positions along the occlusal surface of the fibula. The spheres defined the reference point for measuring implant position. The X, Y, and Z coordinates of each planned and actual implant position were obtained (Figures 5 and 6). The difference in position of the dental implants between the preoperative planned and postoperative actual CT scans was calculated in millimeters.

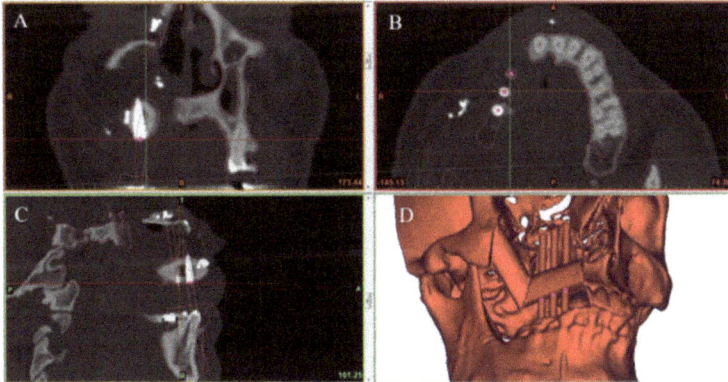

Figure 5. Preoperative CT scan showing virtual planned placement of dental implants in the reconstructed jaw in the (**A**) coronal, (**B**) axial, and (**C**) sagittal planes. (**D**) 3D model showing the final jaw reconstruction with implants in the ideal position according to virtual surgical plan.

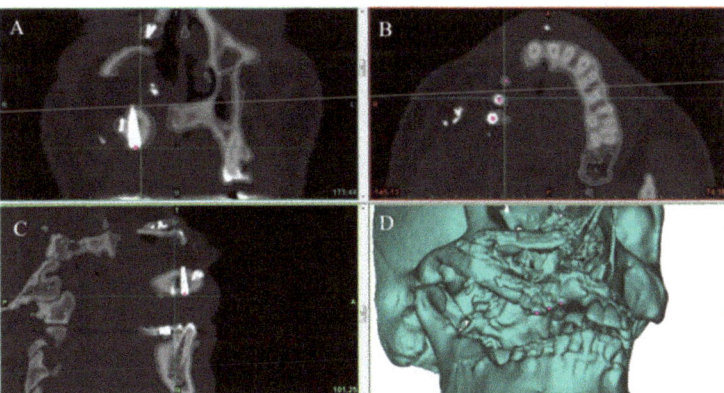

Figure 6. Postoperative CT scan showing the actual position of dental implants in the reconstructed jaw in the (**A**) coronal, (**B**) axial, and (**C**) sagittal planes. (**D**) 3D model showing final jaw reconstruction with implants in their actual position.

3. Results

Patients

Six consecutive patients were included in the analysis. The patient demographics are shown in Table 1. A total of 24 dental implants were inserted, 23 of which were included in the statistical analysis. One implant was inserted at the time of the first stage of surgery but was not planned using SDS and was excluded from our analysis. All flaps survived, there was no implant loss postoperatively, and all the patients that underwent all stages of the reconstruction maintained functional and stable occlusion.

Table 1. Demographics.

Patient	Age (Years)	Sex	Diagnosis	Jaw Defect
1	46	F	Ameloblastoma	Maxilla
2	27	M	Hemangioma	Maxilla
3	61	M	SCC	Maxilla
4	23	M	Ameloblastoma	Mandible
5	49	M	Keratocyst	Maxilla
6	56	F	ORN	Maxilla

F: female; M: male; ORN: osteoradionecrosis; SCC: squamous cell carcinoma.

When the postoperative scans were superimposed on the preoperative SDS plans, the mean center-point distances between the actual and planned implant positions were 1.5 mm (SD ± 1.2 mm) in the X axis, 2.0 mm (SD ± 1.0 mm) in the Y axis, and 1.8 mm (SD ± 1.1 mm) in the Z axis (Figure 7).

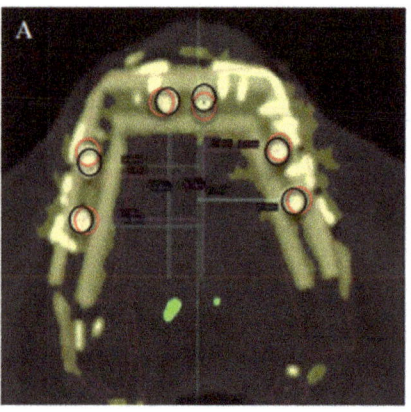
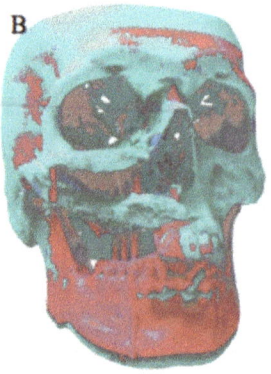

Figure 7. (A) Superimposition of the planned (black circles) dental implant locations according to virtual reconstruction planning and actual (red circles) implant locations on the postoperative CT. (B) Registration of the preoperative 3D model and the postoperative 3D reconstruction, showing overall deviation from the virtual plan.

4. Discussion

This study examined the accuracy of the SDS workflow and AM modifications of fibular flap prefabrication in a cohort of patients undergoing jaw reconstructions. The mean deviations in implant positions from the virtual surgical plans were 1.5, 2.0, and 1.8 mm in the X, Y, and Z axes, respectively. Our findings suggest that the use of SDS in planning osseointegrated dental implants in the prefabricated fibula achieves spatially accurate results in patients undergoing jaw reconstruction. In addition, the minor deviations seen in our cohort were not clinically significant, as they could easily be accommodated for in the final prosthesis. Specifically, all patients in the study developed and maintained good functional occlusion.

Our findings are supported by evidence in the literature. Schepers et al. [13] evaluated the accuracy of placement of fibular grafts and dental implants compared to a virtual plan during a one-stage procedure involving the immediate installation of dental implants. They found a mean deviation of 3.3 mm between the virtually planned implants and the postoperative implants [13].

The use of vascularized bone free flaps has improved the functional and aesthetic outcomes of osseous reconstructions [14,15]. The fibula flap most similarly resembles the jaw, both dimensionally and biomechanically [16,17]. This similarity is why we chose to assess the fibula free flap for our study and is why the fibula free flap is used in our routine practice in caring for patients requiring reconstruction of the jaw for similar defects. The fibula provides excellent bone stock, good soft tissue components, and has a long pedicle that has good caliber vessels for anastomosis [18,19]. The fibula is composed of strong bicortical bone, offering increased primary stability to an implant that is superior to other donor sites [14,15,17,20–24]. Furthermore, the bone can be further augmented by impacting the marrow of the donor fibula with demineralized bone or morselized fibular bone, resulting in improved implant longevity [25,26].

This study reports the clinical accuracy of SDS for osseointegrated implant positioning in prefabricated fibular free flap procedures. We showed that the use of SDS and personalized patient plans improve accuracy of osteointegrated implants and potentially may improve the patients' functional and cosmetic outcomes after jaw reconstruction. The study had some limitations because it was a single-center study and, therefore, susceptible to biases of such a design. Furthermore, the sample size was small so the results must be interpreted with caution.

5. Conclusions

SDS planning of fibular flap prefabrication resulted in better than 2 mm accuracy of osteointegrated implant placement in a cohort of patients undergoing jaw reconstruction. This accuracy could potentially result in improved functional and cosmetic outcomes

Author Contributions: Conceptualization, S.I., H.L., P.T., M.O., S.N. and H.S.; methodology, S.I., H.L., P.T., M.O., S.N. and H.S.; software, S.I. and H.L.; formal analysis, S.I., H.L., P.T., M.O., S.N. and H.S; data curation, S.I., H.L. and P.T.; writing—original draft preparation, S.I., H.L. and P.T.; writing—critical review and editing, S.I., H.L., P.T., M.O., S.N. and H.S. All authors have read and agreed to the published version of the manuscript.

Funding: This research received no external funding.

Institutional Review Board Statement: The study was conducted in accordance with the Declaration of Helsinki, and approved by the Ethics Committee of University of Alberta Health Research Ethics Board (Pro00096288, 26 November 2019).

Informed Consent Statement: Informed consent was obtained from all subjects involved in the study.

Data Availability Statement: The data presented in this study are available on request from the corresponding author. The data are not publicly available due to privacy and ethical restrictions.

Conflicts of Interest: The authors declare no conflict of interest.

References

1. Rohner, D.; Jaquiéry, C.; Kunz, C.; Bucher, P.; Maas, H.; Hammer, B. Maxillofacial reconstruction with prefabricated osseous free flaps: A 3-year experience with 24 patients. *Plast. Reconstr. Surg.* **2003**, *112*, 748–757. [CrossRef] [PubMed]
2. Weitz, J.; Bauer, F.J.M.; Hapfelmeier, A.; Rohleder, N.H.; Wolff, K.D.; Kesting, M.R. Accuracy of mandibular reconstruction by three-dimensional guided vascularised fibular free flap after segmental mandibulectomy. *J. Maxillofac. Oral Surg.* **2016**, *54*, 506–510. [CrossRef] [PubMed]
3. Toto, J.M.; Chang, E.I.; Agag, R.; Devarajan, K.; Patel, S.A.; Topham, N.S. Improved operative efficiency of free fibula flap mandible reconstruction with patient-specific, computer-guided preoperative planning. *Head Neck* **2015**, *37*, 1660–1664. [CrossRef] [PubMed]

4. Hanasono, M.M.; Weinstock, Y.E.; Yu, P. Reconstruction of extensive head and neck defects with multiple simultaneous free flaps. *Plast. Reconstr. Surg.* **2008**, *122*, 1739–1746. [CrossRef]
5. Seruya, M.; Fisher, M.; Rodriguez, E.D. Computer-assisted versus conventional free fibula flap technique for craniofacial reconstruction. *Plast. Reconstr. Surg.* **2013**, *132*, 1219–1228. [CrossRef]
6. Wu, J.; Sun, J.; Shen, S.G.; Xu, B.; Li, J.; Zhang, S. Computer-assisted navigation: Its role in intraoperatively accurate mandibular reconstruction. *Oral Surg. Oral Med. Oral Pathol. Oral Radiol.* **2016**, *122*, 134–142. [CrossRef]
7. Ochi, M.; Kanazawa, M.; Sato, D.; Kasugai, S.; Hirano, S.; Minakuchi, S. Factors affecting accuracy of implant placement with mucosa-supported stereolithographic surgical guides in edentulous mandibles. *Comput. Biol. Med.* **2013**, *43*, 1653–1660. [CrossRef]
8. Zhang, N.; Liu, S.; Hu, Z.; Hu, J.; Zhu, S.; Li, Y. Accuracy of virtual surgical planning in two-jaw orthognathic surgery: Comparison of planned and actual results. *Oral Surg. Oral Med. Oral Pathol. Oral Radiol.* **2016**, *122*, 143–151. [CrossRef]
9. Okay, D.J.; Buchbinder, D.; Urken, M.; Jacobson, A.; Lazarus, C.; Persky, M. Computer-assisted implant rehabilitation of maxillomandibular defects reconstructed with vascularized bone free flaps. *JAMA Otolaryngol. Head Neck Surg.* **2013**, *139*, 371–381. [CrossRef]
10. Toro, C.; Robiony, M.; Costa, F.; Zerman, N.; Politi, M. Feasibility of preoperative planning using anatomical facsimile models for mandibular reconstruction. *Head Face Med.* **2007**, *3*, 1006–1011. [CrossRef]
11. Zheng, G.-S.; Su, Y.-X.; Liao, G.-Q.; Liu, H.-C.; Zhang, S.-E.; Liang, L.-Z. Mandibular reconstruction assisted by preoperative simulation and accurate transferring templates: Preliminary report of clinical application. *J. Oral Maxillofac. Surg.* **2013**, *71*, 1613–1618. [CrossRef] [PubMed]
12. Seikaly, H.; Idris, S.; Chuka, R.; Jeffrey, C.; Dzioba, A.; Makki, F.; Logan, H.; O'Connell, D.A.; Harris, J.; Ansari, K.; et al. The Alberta Reconstructive Technique: An occlusion-driven and digitally based jaw reconstruction. *Laryngoscope* **2019**, *129*, S1–S14. [CrossRef] [PubMed]
13. Schepers, R.H.; Raghoebar, G.M.; Vissink, A.; Stenekes, M.W.; Kraeima, J.; Roodenburgm, J.L.; Reintsema, H.; Witjes, M.J. Accuracy of fibula reconstruction using patient-specific CAD/CAM reconstruction plates and dental implants: A new modality for functional reconstruction of mandibular defects. *J. Craniomaxillofac. Surg.* **2015**, *43*, 649–657. [CrossRef] [PubMed]
14. Avraham, T.; Franco, P.; Brecht, L.E.; Ceradini, D.J.; Saadeh, P.B.; Hirsch, D.L.; Levine, J.P. Functional outcomes of virtually planned free fibula flap reconstruction of the mandible. *Plast. Reconstr. Surg.* **2014**, *134*, 628e–6234e. [CrossRef] [PubMed]
15. Kramer, F.J.; Dempf, R.; Bremer, B. Efficacy of dental implants placed into fibula-free flaps for orofacial reconstruction. *Clin. Oral Implants Res.* **2005**, *16*, 80–88. [CrossRef] [PubMed]
16. Seikaly, H.; Chau, J.; Li, F.; Driscoll, B.; Seikaly, D.; Calhoun, J.; Calhoun, K.H. Bone that best matches the properties of the mandible. *J. Otolaryngol.* **2003**, *32*, 262–265. [CrossRef] [PubMed]
17. Ide, Y.; Matsunaga, S.; Harris, J.; O'Connell, D.; Seikaly, H.; Wolfaardt, J. Anatomical examination of the fibula: Digital imaging study for osseointegrated implant installation. *J. Otolaryngol. Head Neck Surg.* **2015**, *44*, 1. [CrossRef]
18. Hidalgo, D.A. Fibula free flap. *Plast. Reconstr. Surg.* **1989**, *84*, 71–79. [CrossRef]
19. Hayden, R.E.; Mullin, D.P.; Patel, A.K. Reconstruction of the segmental mandibular defect. *Curr. Opin. Otolaryngol. Head Neck Surg.* **2012**, *20*, 231–236. [CrossRef]
20. Matsuurra, M.; Ohno, K.; Michi, K.; Egawa, K.; Takiguchi, R. Clinicoanatomic examination of the fibula: Anatomic basis for dental implant placement. *Int. J. Oral Maxillofac. Implants* **1999**, *14*, 879–884.
21. Niimil, A.; Ozekil, K.; Uedal, M.; Nakayama, B. A comparative study of removal torque of endosseous implants in the fibula, iliac crest and scapula of cadavers: Preliminary report. *Clin. Oral Implants Res.* **1997**, *8*, 286–289. [CrossRef] [PubMed]
22. Ivanoff, C.J.; Sennerby, L.; Lekholm, U. Influence of mono- and bicortical anchorage on the integration of titanium implants. *Int. J. Oral Maxillofac. Surg.* **1996**, *25*, 229–235. [CrossRef]
23. Seikaly, H.; Maharaj, M.; Rieger, J.; Harris, J. Functional outcomes after primary mandibular resection and reconstruction with the fibular free flap. *J. Otolaryngol.* **2005**, *34*, 25–28. [CrossRef] [PubMed]
24. Logan, H.; Wolfaardt, J.; Boulanger, P.; Hodgetts, B.; Seikaly, H. Exploratory benchtop study evaluating the use of surgical design and simulation in fibula free flap mandibular reconstruction. *J. Otolaryngol. Head Neck Surg.* **2013**, *42*, 42. [CrossRef]
25. Barber, B.R.; Dziegelewski, P.T.; Chuka, R.; O'Connell, D.; Harris, J.R.; Seikaly, H. Bone-impacted fibular free flap: Long-term dental implant success and complications compared to traditional fibular free tissue transfer. *Head Neck* **2015**, *38* (Suppl. S1), E1783–E1787. [CrossRef]
26. Dziegielewski, P.T.; Mlynarek, A.M.; Harris, J.R.; Hrdlicka, A.; Barber, B.; Al-Qahtani, K.; Wolfaardt, J.; Raboud, D.; Seikaly, H. Bone impacted fibular free flap: A novel technique to increase bone density for dental implantation in osseous reconstruction. *Head Neck* **2013**, *36*, 1648–1653. [CrossRef]

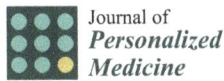

Article

A Two-Step Approach for 3D-Guided Patient-Specific Corrective Limb Osteotomies

Nick Assink [1,2,*], Anne M. L. Meesters [1,2], Kaj ten Duis [2], Jorrit S. Harbers [2], Frank F. A. IJpma [2], Hugo C. van der Veen [3], Job N. Doornberg [3], Peter A. J. Pijpker [1,3] and Joep Kraeima [1]

1. 3D Lab, University Medical Centre Groningen, University of Groningen, 9713 GZ Groningen, The Netherlands
2. Department of Surgery, University Medical Centre Groningen, University of Groningen, 9713 GZ Groningen, The Netherlands
3. Department of Orthopaedic Surgery, University Medical Centre Groningen, University of Groningen, 9713 GZ Groningen, The Netherlands
* Correspondence: n.assink@umcg.nl

Abstract: *Background:* Corrective osteotomy surgery for long bone anomalies can be very challenging since deformation of the bone is often present in three dimensions. We developed a two-step approach for 3D-planned corrective osteotomies which consists of a cutting and reposition guide in combination with a conventional osteosynthesis plate. This study aimed to assess accuracy of the achieved corrections using this two-step technique. *Methods:* All patients (≥12 years) treated for post-traumatic malunion with a two-step 3D-planned corrective osteotomy within our center in 2021 were prospectively included. Three-dimensional virtual models of the planned outcome and the clinically achieved outcome were obtained and aligned. Postoperative evaluation of the accuracy of performed corrections was assessed by measuring the preoperative and postoperative alignment error in terms of angulation, rotation and translation. *Results:* A total of 10 patients were included. All corrective osteotomies were performed according to the predetermined surgical plan without any complications. The preoperative deformities ranged from 7.1 to 27.5° in terms of angulation and 5.3 to 26.1° in terms of rotation. The achieved alignment deviated on average 2.1 ± 1.0 and 3.4 ± 1.6 degrees from the planning for the angulation and rotation, respectively. *Conclusions:* A two-step approach for 3D-guided patient-specific corrective limb osteotomies is reliable, feasible and accurate.

Keywords: virtual surgical planning; 3D printing; 3D technology; three-dimensional; corrective osteotomy; osteotomies; malunion; patient-specific; patient-specific instruments; surgical guide

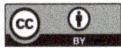

1. Introduction

Corrective osteotomy surgery for long bone anomalies can be very challenging since the deformation of the bone is often present in three dimensions. Conventional planning methods use two-dimensional (2D) imaging to plan the osteotomy and subsequent surgery is performed freehand, which leads to unpredictable results. With rapid advances in three-dimensional (3D) printing technologies, surgeons have started to apply 3D printing for a wide range of applications in orthopedic trauma surgery [1]. Particularly in corrective osteotomy surgery, the use of 3D-printed surgical guides is well-described and shows promising results in terms of functional outcome and reduced operating time [1–4]. The use of 3D virtual surgical planning allows the surgeon to visualize the anatomy in 3D, and virtually plan the osteotomy based on the CT scan. Additionally, patient-specific instruments can be designed and 3D printed to guide the cutting and reduction process during surgery. This process takes into account the specific anatomy of the patient and the desired surgical approach, which might lead to a more accurate result [5].

In recent years, different respective methods and techniques for corrective osteotomies of various mechanisms of deformities (i.e., post-traumatic deformities, growth disturbances, congenital anomalies) have been described. The majority of these methods consist of a surgical guide with a cutting slot for the planned osteotomy plane and drilling holes for preplanned screws [6–12]. Since the screw holes are predrilled, this technique requires an adequate fit of the preplanned plate in order to achieve the planned correction. However, due to the deformity of the bone, conventional plates usually do not fit, which potentially compromises accuracy and can lead to impaired functional outcome. For some cases, precontouring the plate provides a solution [11]. However, bending of a plate does not always result in a good fit; therefore, another solution for adequate use of this 3D technology may be provided by using a patient-specific plate [12]. Yet, currently, patient-specific plates are not widely available; they may be costly and pose logistical and legal challenges. An alternative reported approach is the use of a surgical cutting guide in combination with a reduction guide. The correction is then controlled by placing Kirschner wires (K-wires) with the cutting guide and subsequently realigning of the K-wires towards a parallel position with the use of a reduction guide. However, the combined use of both a reduction guide and a plate is often limited by the small surgical working space. This technique is only described for a few applications [13–16].

We present this alternative strategy, which consists of our two-step approach for 3D-planned corrective osteotomy, which has been successfully clinically applied. Our method adds to previous reports because a reduction guide, which envelops the planned osteosynthesis plate, is introduced, and therefore the technique is less limited by the surgical working space. This method can be applied disregarding the deformation or location, and is based on our experience in 3D-planned corrective osteotomy surgery over the past few years. This study aimed to assess the accuracy of the achieved corrections using this technique.

2. Materials and Methods

2.1. Patients

All patients ($\geq$12 years) treated for post-traumatic malunion with a single- or double-cut 3D-planned corrective osteotomy within our center between January and December 2021 were prospectively included upon availability of a pre- and postoperative CT scan with a slice thickness of less than 1 mm. The institutional review board of our center approved the study procedures, and the research was performed in accordance with the relevant guidelines and regulations (registry: 202100639). Written consent was obtained from all patients.

2.2. 3D Virtual Surgical Planning of the Corrective Osteotomy

For all patients, a CT scan of the malunited as well as the corresponding contralateral uninjured bone was available. The DICOM (Digital Imaging and Communications in Medicine) image data were imported into the Mimics Medical software package (Version 21.0, Materialise, Leuven, Belgium) in order to create a 3D reconstruction of the affected bone and its counterpart. A segmentation process was performed using a preset bone threshold (Hounsfield unit $\geq$ 226) combined with the 'region growing' and 'split mask' function in order to separate the bone from adjacent bones. After the segmentation process, the 3D models of both the malunited and the contralateral bone were imported into the 3-matic software (Version 15.0, Materialise, Leuven, Belgium). The contralateral bone was then mirrored and aligned on an unaffected part of the malunited bone in order to measure the deviation. Based on the deviation, the osteotomy and correction were planned, and a virtual model of the osteosynthesis plate chosen by the surgeon was imported and positioned on the corrected bone. K-wires, at least two on each side of the osteotomy plane, were then placed parallel on the bone after virtual correction, duplicated and reversed engineered towards their original position on the 'uncorrected' malunited bone. A cutting guide was then designed, which included the planned osteotomy and the position of the K-wires before correction. In addition, a reposition guide was designed to be placed on top of the planned plate, fitting the K-wires as positioned after the planned correction

(Figure 1). During this workflow, multiple interdisciplinary meetings between technical physicians and (orthopedic) trauma surgeons were held to determine surgical approach, level of osteotomy and desired plate positioning in order to ultimately meet our patient's clinical needs.

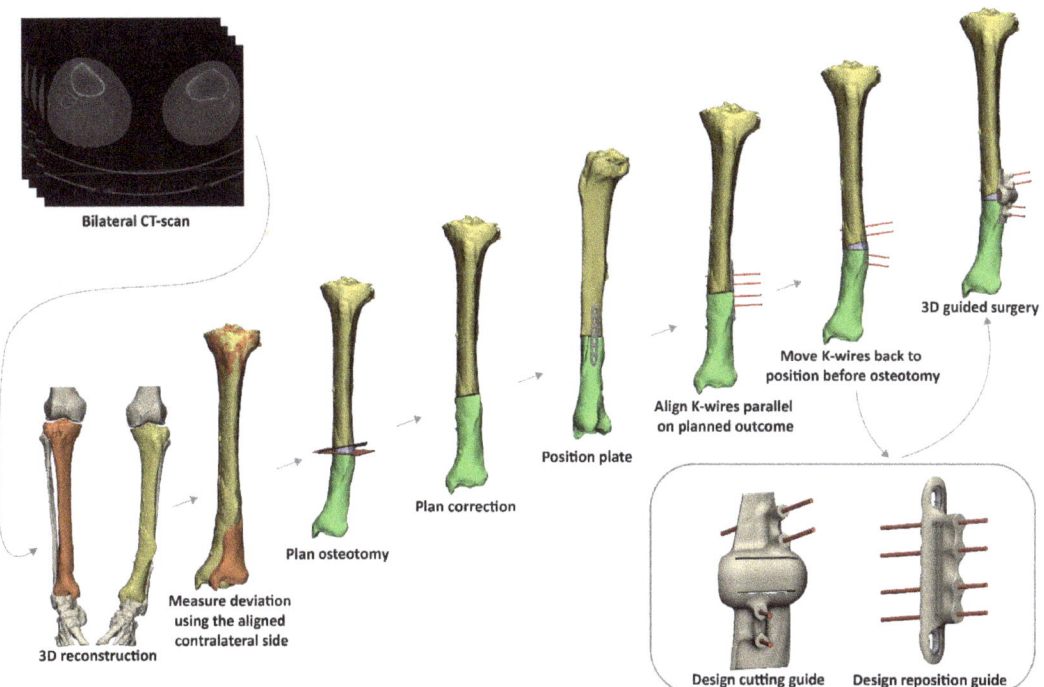

Figure 1. Workflow of a 3D-guided patient-specific corrective osteotomy using a two-step approach. (1) First, a 3D reconstruction is made from a bilateral CT scan. (2) By mirroring and aligning the contralateral (healthy) side on the malunited bone (orange), the deviation is measured. (3) Based on the deviation, the osteotomy and the correction are planned. (4) An osteosynthesis plate is chosen and positioned on the bone after correction. (5) K-wires are positioned parallel on the planned correction. (6) K-wires are placed parallel on the corrected bone, duplicated and moved to the corresponding position on the malunited bone before the correction is performed. (7) Patient-specific cutting and reposition guides are designed. (8) 3D-guided osteotomy is performed using the patient-specific cutting guide. Subsequently, the cutting guide is removed and the reposition guide (including the plate) is slid over the K-wires to achieve the intended correction.

2.3. Surgical Procedure

After designing the guides, the patient-specific cutting and reposition guides were 3D-printed by selective laser sintering using polyamide 12 (PA12). Additionally, real-size models of the malunion and planned correction were printed 1:1. These prints were sterilized and used during surgery. Exposure of the affected bone was obtained during surgery using a surgical approach as discussed with the surgeon during the stepwise 3D planning process. The cutting guide was then fitted on the bone using bony landmarks, and the K-wires were then placed through the guide (Figures 2c and 3c). The unique footprint directs the guide to the intended location. Positioning of the guide was confirmed by verifying the position of the K-wires with respect to the bony landmarks using fluoroscopy. In the case of incorrect positioning, the guide was repositioned until the surgeon was confident about the correct positioning after repeated visual inspection and radiographic confirmation. The osteotomy was performed through the cutting slot of the cutting guide using an oscillating saw. Subsequently, the planned correction was performed by aligning the K-wires to a parallel position. This process was controlled by sliding the reposition guide, which enveloped the plate, over the K-wires (Figures 2d and 3d). In opening-wedge high tibial osteotomy cases, the planned wedge was incorporated into the guide design for additional strength of the construct and to prevent K-wires from bending during the opening of the wedge (Figure 3). After correction, the design of the reposition guide allowed for at least two screws to be drilled and placed both distal and proximal to the osteotomy level. After placement of these screws, the reposition guide was removed, and the remaining screws were placed. The reposition guide was designed in such a way that the construct of the guide with the fixed K-wires did not block the drilling and placement of the screws.

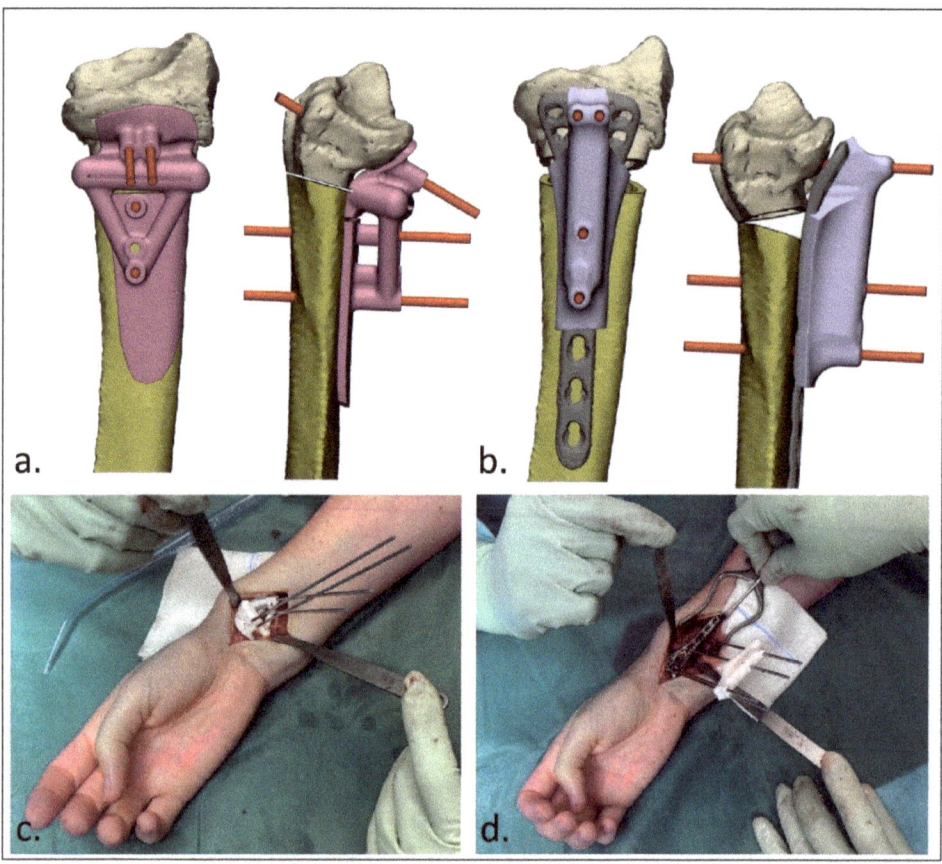

Figure 2. 3D-guided patient-specific corrective osteotomy of a malunited distal radius that was initially treated conservatively in a cast (Case 6). (**a**) Frontal and lateral view of the designed cutting guide (pink) with the -wires (red); (**b**) frontal and lateral view of the designed reposition guide (purple) with the parallel K-wires (red); (**c**) operative usage of the cutting guide; (**d**) operative usage of the reposition guide. The specific design of the reposition guide allowed for at least two screws to be drilled and placed both distal and proximal to the osteotomy level. Note the convergent K-wires in the cutting guide (**c**), and the parallel K-wires as reduction aids in the reposition guide (**d**).

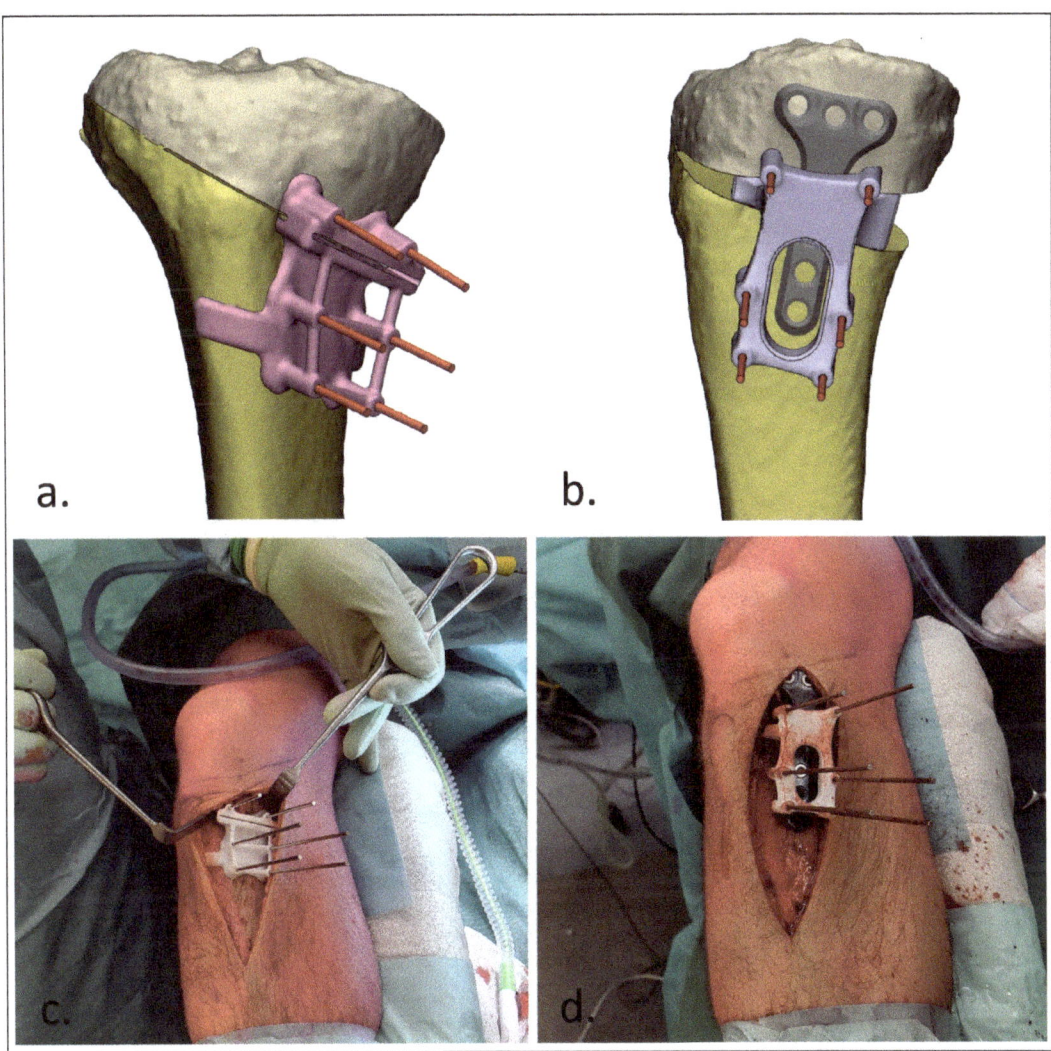

Figure 3. 3D-guided patient-specific corrective osteotomy of a proximal tibia (Case 8). (**a**) Frontal view of the designed cutting guide (pink) with the K-wires; (**b**) lateral view of the designed reposition guide (purple) with the parallel K-wires and insertion of the planned wedge; (**c**) operative usage of the cutting guide; (**d**) operative usage of the reposition guide.

2.4. Postoperative Evaluation

Postoperative evaluation of the accuracy of the performed correction was performed by superimposition of the plan and the postoperative outcome. Subsequently, the preoperative and postoperative alignment error were measured in terms of angulation, rotation and translation. A 3D model of the bone before correction was retrieved from the initial planning. This model was duplicated and aligned with the planned outcome and the postoperative 3D model, such that there were three identical parts with different alignments (preoperative, planned and postoperative parts). In order to measure the angulation and rotation, the inertia axes were automatically drawn using the 'create analytical primitive' function in the 3-matic software (Figure 4a). The angulation was then measured as the difference in angle in the z-axis (Figure 4b) and the rotation as the difference in angle in the x-axis (Figure 4c). The translation was obtained by measuring the Euclidean distance in millimeters between the center of gravity of these three parts (preoperative, planned and postoperative). In addition, the clinical outcome was assessed by evaluating the range of motion before surgery and six months after surgery. A Mann–Whitney U test was performed to assess the difference between planned and obtained angulation, rotation and translation. A p-value of <0.05 was considered statistically significant.

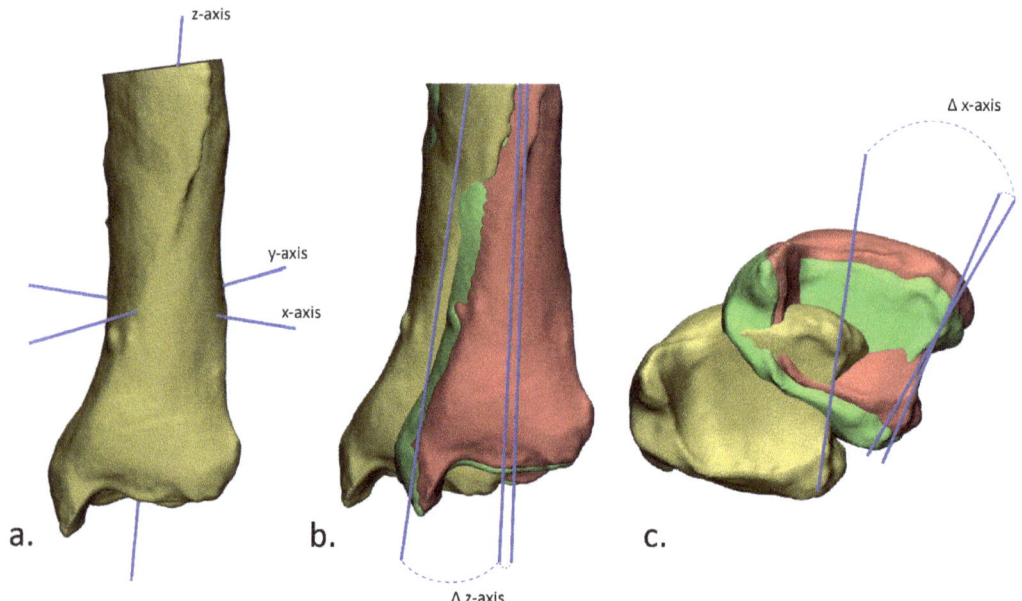

Figure 4. Evaluation of the achieved correction in terms of angulation and rotation. (**a**) First, the inertia axes were determined; (**b**) the angulation was then determined by measuring the angle between the z-axis of the preoperative (yellow) and planned (green) position of the bone, and between the planned and the postoperative (red) position; (**c**) the rotation was determined by measuring the angle between the x-axis of the preoperative and planned position, and the planned and postoperative position.

3. Results

3.1. Patients

A total of 10 patients, treated for their post-traumatic malunion with a 3D-planned corrective osteotomy, were prospectively included in this study. The age of the patients varied from 12 to 64 years old, and seven of the patients were males (Table 1). The patients were treated for a malunion in various bones including the clavicle, humerus, radius, femur and tibia. Indication for corrective osteotomy was loss of function by decreased range of motion post-trauma due to acquired pathoanatomy in all patients with an upper limb deformity ($n = 6$). In the patients with a deformity of the lower limb ($n = 4$), the correction was performed due to complaints of pain and instability of the knee or ankle.

3.2. Accuracy

All corrective osteotomies were performed according to the predetermined plan without any complications. The preoperative deformities ranged from 7.1 to 27.5° in terms of angulation and 5.3 to 26.1° in terms of rotation. The achieved alignment deviated on average 2.1 ± 1.0 and 3.4 ± 1.6 degrees from the planning for the angulation and rotation, respectively (Table 2). In four cases, the achieved angulation was more than what was needed in the planned direction (overcorrection), and in another four cases, the angulation was less than what was needed (undercorrection). In terms of rotation, in four patients, the applied correction was more than intended, whereas in two patients, the correction was less. The achieved positioning of the bone deviated on average 1.8 mm from the intended position. Differences between planned and obtained angulation ($p < 0.001$), rotation ($p = 0.009$) and translation ($p < 0.001$) were found to be statistically significant.

Table 1. Patient characteristics.

	Case	Sex	Age at Time of Surgery (Years)	Area of Deformity	Deformity	Planned Correction
Upper limb	1	F	16	Clavicula	Angulation; Shortening	Closed wedge
	2	F	23	Proximal humerus	Varus; Rotation	Closed wedge
	3	M	12	Midshaft radius	Angulation	Closed wedge
	4	M	16	Distal radius	Rotation	Rotation
	5	M	17	Distal radius	Volar angulation	Open wedge
	6	F	59	Distal radius	Volar angulation	Open wedge
Lower limb	7	M	28	Femur	Rotation	Rotation
	8	M	17	Proximal tibia	Varus; Increased tibial slope	Open wedge
	9	M	24	Proximal tibia	Increased tibial slope	Closed wedge
	10	M	64	Distal tibia	Varus; Rotation	Closed wedge

Table 2. Postoperative evaluation of the performed corrective osteotomies. Accuracy was assessed in terms of angulation (degrees), rotation (degrees) and translation (millimeters).

Case	Angulation (°)			Rotation (°)			Translation (mm)	
	Preoperative vs. Plan	Postoperative vs. Plan	Over/under Correction	Preoperative vs. Plan	Postoperative vs. Plan	Over/under Correction	Preoperative vs. Plan	Postoperative vs. Plan
1	20.5	3.7	Under	-	-	-	8.1	0.3
2	14.7	2.7	Under	22.8	1.3	Over	6.2	3.2
3	14.7	1.3	Over	-	-	-	7.2	0.8
4	-	-	-	26.1	4.3	Over	4.4	0.5
5	12.5	2.7	Over	-	-	-	7.5	1.6
6	27.5	1.8	Over	5.3	1.6	Over	7.1	1.0
7	-	-	-	26.0	5.1	Under	1.1	0.8
8	13.5	2.6	Under	-	-	Over	37.8	6.2
9	7.1	0.2	Under	-	-	-	3.5	0.4
10	13.6	1.6	Over	24.7	4.8	Under	17.2	2.9
Average	15.5 ± 5.7	2.1 ± 1.0		21.0 ± 7.9	3.4 ± 1.6		10.0 ± 10.1	1.8 ± 1.8

3.3. Clinical Outcome

In all six patients who underwent a corrective osteotomy for a malunion of the upper limb, the range of motion was significantly improved after six months (Table 3). After correction of the malunions of the lower limb, all patients reported a significant reduction in pain and instability.

Table 3. Range of motion in the upper extremities before and 6 months after correction.

	Case	Restricted Joint	Preoperative Range of Restricted Motion	Postoperative Range of Motion (6 Months)
Upper limb	1	Clavicula	F/E 110-0-40; Ab/Ad 140-0-30	F/E 160-0-40; Ab/Ad 160-0-30
	2	Proximal humerus	F/E 150-0-40; Ab/Ad: 140-0-30; ER/IR: 90-0-L5	F/E 170-0-40; Ab/Ad: 160-0-30; ER/IR: 80-0-T12
	3	Midshaft radius	P/S: 10-0-60	P/S: 45/0/70
	4	Distal radius	P/S: 70-0-55	P/S: 70-0-80
	5	Distal radius	P/S: 70-0-30	P/S: 70-0-80
	6	Distal radius	F/E: 50/0/20 P/S: 20/0/80	F/E: 40/0/50 P/S: 60/0/80

F/E: flexion/extension, Ab/Ad: abduction/adduction, ER/IR: external rotation/internal rotation, P/S: pronation/supination, L5: 5th lumbar vertebra, T12: 12th thoracic vertebra.

4. Discussion

Bone deformities in both the upper and lower extremities frequently lead to functional impairment, pain, instability and/or aesthetic concerns. Additionally, in the long term, this could lead to early-onset osteoarthritis of adjacent joints. Corrective osteotomy surgery of these post-traumatic acquired deformities can be very challenging since the deformation of the bone is often present in three dimensions. With the use of 3D-printing technologies, corrective osteotomy surgery has become more predictable. In this study, we presented our clinically applied two-step approach (cutting guide followed by reposition guide) of patient-specific 3D-planned corrective limb osteotomies. The results of this study show that our clinically applied method is reliable, feasible, user-friendly and accurate.

Several studies describe 3D-planned corrective limb osteotomies and show their technique to be feasible, leading to good functional outcomes [6–14]. Yet, even though the surgery is planned using state-of-the-art 3D software, postoperative evaluation is usually still performed in 2D on plain radiographs since postoperative CTs are not routinely made. Therefore, the majority of these studies evaluated their achieved accuracy based on postoperative radiographs, thereby only providing the accuracy in two dimensions: the anteroposterior and lateral direction [6–9,11]. Since the performed correction was planned in three dimensions, it is essential to assess the postoperative result in three dimensions as well to provide the accuracy of the performed correction and to gain insight into the cause of deviation in relation to suboptimal clinical outcomes. Omori et al. performed corrective osteotomies in 17 patients with a deformity of the humerus and compared postoperative 3D bone models with the preoperative planning using a surface registration technique [13]. In terms of translation, they showed a mean error of 1.7 mm in anterior–posterior translation, 1.3 mm in lateral–medial translation and 7.1 mm in proximal–distal translation, whereas they showed mean errors of 0.6°, 0.8° and 2.9° for varus–valgus, flexion–extension and internal–external rotation, respectively. Additionally, Dobbe et al. successfully performed a 3D-guided corrective osteotomy using a patient-specific plate in seven patients with post-traumatic distal radius deformities and showed a median residual translation and rotation error of 3.0 mm and 8.5°, respectively [12]. In addition to these scarce studies, this current study is one of the few studies which assessed the postoperative result in 3D. Where the previous studies were limited to one specific malunited bone, in this study, we performed 3D-planned corrective limb osteotomies in different body regions of ten patients, indicating the wide applicability of our technique. The results of this study show similar accuracy compared to previous reports with an average angulation of $2.1 \pm 1.0°$, rotation of $3.4 \pm 1.6°$ and translation of 1.8 ± 1.8 mm.

The rationale behind using patient-specific 3D-printed guides is that it helps the surgeon perform the osteotomy and predrill the screws more reliably and according to the plan, leading to a more accurate correction. However, one of the possible pitfalls is translation of bone fragments over the osteotomy planes due to applied uncontrolled compression on the plate [10]. This is especially true in cases with extensive deformation of the bone where there is no good fit between the plate and bone. A suboptimal correction in these patients may result in residual functional impairment, pain and joint instability. Our two-step approach provides a solution for these patients by not predrilling the screws but using K-wires to secure the cutting guide, and subsequentially a reposition guide with these positioned K-wires, which forces bone fragments into the correct 3D-planned alignment while serving as a temporary fixation as well. The plate can generally be placed under the reposition guide for easy application. The specific design of the reposition guide allows for at least two screws to be drilled and placed both distal and proximal to the osteotomy level, which then hold the reposition while the guide is removed. Definitive fixation can then be performed by placing the remaining screws within the plate.

One of the limitations of this pilot study is the relatively small patient group. Since the goal of this study was to critically evaluate the accuracy of our two-step approach, we included all patients who were treated with this technique irrespective of anatomical site or nature of the post-traumatic deformity. Even though this study showed that our technique is clinically feasible and accurate in both upper and lower extremity deformities, the inclusion of different osteotomy locations led to a highly heterogeneous study population. Yet, one could also argue this a study strength, as it improves the external validity of our results regardless of the anatomical site. Additionally, since the primary aim of this research was to assess the accuracy of this technique, the clinical outcome in this study was limited to the range of motion, which was only of importance in the cases with upper limb deformities. Further studies should also incorporate patient-reported outcomes to also fully assess the impact of this method on functional recovery. This is especially true in patients with lower limb deformities, since these patients were not affected by a restricted range of motion.

Even though high accuracy of the planned correction was achieved in all patients, some minimal residual angulation, rotation and translation error were still present, although we argue this is clinically not relevant to patients' functional outcome. At this stage, it is impossible to assess at what part of the surgery the error happened (e.g., positioning of the guides, securing the screws). In order to further improve the current method, it would be recommended to investigate each specific step within the procedure. In particular, the positioning of the cutting guide along the longitudinal axis is usually quite challenging in the case anatomical landmarks for verifying the correct position of the guides are limited (e.g., shaft fractures). Where the proximal or distal end of the bone generally has quite distinguishable features, the fit of the guide on the midshaft bone is usually less rigid. Further investigation on what impact guide positioning has on the accuracy is therefore recommended. In addition, this study included patients with relatively severe deformities with an average angulation of $15.5 \pm 5.7°$ and rotation of $21.0 \pm 7.9°$. Patients with more subtle deformities might also benefit from 3D-guided corrective osteotomy surgery. To our knowledge, no clear cut-off for the point at which a deformity is too small to correct accurately has been established. Therefore, it further investigation of what deformities can accurately be corrected in order to utilize this technique to its full potential is also recommended.

5. Conclusions

This study showed that a two-step approach for 3D-guided patient-specific corrective limb osteotomies is reliable, feasible, user-friendly and accurate for corrective osteotomies of deformities of all long bones.

Author Contributions: Conceptualization: N.A., A.M.L.M., P.A.J.P. and J.K.; Methodology: N.A., A.M.L.M., P.A.J.P. and J.K.; Software: N.A., A.M.L.M., P.A.J.P. and J.K.; Validation: N.A., A.M.L.M., K.t.D., J.S.H., F.F.A.I., H.C.v.d.V., J.N.D., P.A.J.P. and J.K.; Formal analysis: N.A., A.M.L.M., K.t.D., J.S.H., F.F.A.I., H.C.v.d.V., J.N.D., P.A.J.P. and J.K.; Investigation: N.A., A.M.L.M., K.t.D., J.S.H., F.F.A.I.,

H.C.v.d.V., J.N.D., P.A.J.P. and J.K.; Resources: K.t.D., J.S.H., F.F.A.I., H.C.v.d.V., J.N.D. and J.K.; Data curation: N.A., A.M.L.M. and P.A.J.P.; Writing—original draft preparation: N.A., A.M.L.M. and P.A.J.P.; Writing—review and editing: K.t.D., J.S.H., F.F.A.I., H.C.v.d.V., J.N.D. and J.K.; Visualization: N.A.; Supervision: J.K.; Project administration: N.A.; Funding acquisition: Not Applicable. All authors have read and agreed to the published version of the manuscript.

Funding: This research received no external funding.

Institutional Review Board Statement: The study was conducted according to the guidelines of the Declaration of Helsinki, and approved by the Institutional Review Board of the University Medical Centre Groningen (registry: 202100639; date of approval: 8 November 2021).

Informed Consent Statement: Informed consent was obtained from all subjects involved in the study.

Data Availability Statement: The authors declare that the data supporting the findings of this study are available within the paper.

Conflicts of Interest: The authors declare no conflict of interest.

References

1. Lal, H.; Patralekh, M.K. 3D printing and its applications in orthopaedic trauma: A technological marvel. *J. Clin. Orthop. Trauma* **2018**, *9*, 260–268. [CrossRef] [PubMed]
2. Tack, P.; Victor, J.; Gemmel, P.; Annemans, L. 3D-printing techniques in a medical setting: A systematic literature review. *Biomed. Eng. Online* **2016**, *15*, 115. [CrossRef] [PubMed]
3. Baraza, N.; Chapman, C.; Zakani, S.; Mulpuri, K. 3D-printed patient specific instrumentation in corrective osteotomy of the femur and pelvis: A review of the literature. *3D Print Med.* **2020**, *6*, 34. [CrossRef] [PubMed]
4. Raza, M.; Murphy, D.; Gelfer, Y. The effect of three-dimensional (3D) printing on quantitative and qualitative outcomes in paediatric orthopaedic osteotomies: A systematic review. *EFORT Open Rev.* **2021**, *6*, 130–138. [CrossRef] [PubMed]
5. Hoekstra, H.; Rosseels, W.; Sermon, A.; Nijs, S. Corrective limb osteotomy using patient specific 3D-printed guides: A technical note. *Injury* **2016**, *47*, 2375–2380. [CrossRef] [PubMed]
6. Buijze, G.A.; Leong, N.L.; Stockmans, F.; Axelsson, P.; Moreno, R.; Sörensen, A.I.; Jupiter, J.B. Three-dimensional compared with two-dimensional preoperative planning of corrective osteotomy for extra-articular distal radial malunion: A multicenter randomized controlled trial. *J. Bone Jt. Surg. Am.* **2018**, *100*, 1191–1202. [CrossRef] [PubMed]
7. Michielsen, M.; van Haver, A.; Bertrand, V.; Vanhees, M.; Verstreken, F. Corrective osteotomy of distal radius malunions using three-dimensional computer simulation and patient-specific guides to achieve anatomic reduction. *Eur. J. Orthop. Surg. Traumatol.* **2018**, *28*, 1531–1535. [CrossRef] [PubMed]
8. Athlani, L.; Chenel, A.; Detammaecker, R.; de Almeida, Y.-K.; Dautel, G. Computer-assisted 3D preoperative planning of corrective osteotomy for extra-articular distal radius malunion: A 16-patient case series. *Hand Surg. Rehabil.* **2020**, *39*, 275–283. [CrossRef] [PubMed]
9. Oka, K.; Tanaka, H.; Okada, K.; Sahara, W.; Myoui, A.; Yamada, T.; Yamamoto, M.; Kurimoto, S.; Hirata, H.; Murase, T. Three-dimensional corrective osteotomy for malunited fractures of the upper extremity using patient-matched instruments: A prospective, multicenter, open-label, single-arm trial. *J. Bone Jt. Surg. Am.* **2019**, *101*, 710–721. [CrossRef] [PubMed]
10. Rosseels, W.; Herteleer, M.; Sermon, A.; Nijs, S.; Hoekstra, H. Corrective osteotomies using patient-specific 3D-printed guides: A critical appraisal. *Eur. J. Trauma Emerg. Surg.* **2019**, *45*, 299–307. [CrossRef] [PubMed]
11. Roth, K.C.; van Es, E.M.; Kraan, G.A.; Verhaar, J.A.N.; Stockmans, F.; Colaris, J.W. Outcomes of 3-D corrective osteotomies for paediatric malunited both-bone forearm fractures. *J. Hand Surg.* **2022**, *47*, 164–171. [CrossRef] [PubMed]
12. Dobbe, J.G.G.; Peymani, A.; Roos, H.A.L.; Beerens, M.; Streekstra, G.J.; Strackee, S.D. Patient-specific plate for navigation and fixation of the distal radius: A case series. *Int. J. Comput. Assist. Radiol. Surg.* **2021**, *16*, 515–524. [CrossRef] [PubMed]
13. Omori, S.; Murase, T.; Oka, K.; Kawanishi, Y.; Oura, K.; Tanaka, H.; Yoshikawa, H. Postoperative accuracy analysis of three-dimensional corrective osteotomy for cubitus varus deformity with a custom-made surgical guide based on computer simulation. *J. Shoulder Elbow Surg.* **2015**, *24*, 242–249. [CrossRef] [PubMed]
14. Bauer, D.E.; Zimmermann, S.; Aichmair, A.; Hingsammer, A.; Schweizer, A.; Nagy, L.; Fürnstahl, P. Conventional versus computer-assisted corrective osteotomy of the forearm: A retrospective analysis of 56 consecutive cases. *J. Hand Surg. Am.* **2017**, *42*, 447–455. [CrossRef] [PubMed]
15. Gerbers, J.G.; Pijpker, P.A.J.; Brouwer, R.W.; van der Veen, H.C. Anterolateral proximal tibial opening wedge osteotomy for biplanar correction in genu valgum recurvatum using patient specific instrumentation (PSI). A technical note. *Knee* **2021**, *33*, 58–64. [CrossRef] [PubMed]
16. van Raaij, T.; van der Wel, H.; Beldman, M.; de Vries, A.; Kraeima, J. Two-Step 3D-Guided Supramalleolar Osteotomy to Treat Varus Ankle osteoarthritis. *Foot Ankle Int.* **2022**, *43*, 937–941. [CrossRef] [PubMed]

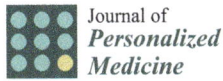

Article

Quantitative Three-Dimensional Measurements of Acetabular Fracture Displacement Could Be Predictive for Native Hip Survivorship [†]

Anne M. L. Meesters [1,2], Miriam G. E. Oldhoff [1,2], Neeltje M. Trouwborst [1], Nick Assink [1,2], Joep Kraeima [2,3], Max J. H. Witjes [2,3], Jean-Paul P. M. de Vries [1], Kaj ten Duis [1] and Frank F. A. IJpma [1,*]

1. Department of Surgery, University Medical Center Groningen, University of Groningen, 9713 GZ Groningen, The Netherlands
2. 3D Lab, University Medical Center Groningen, University of Groningen, 9713 GZ Groningen, The Netherlands
3. Department of Oral and Maxillofacial Surgery, University Medical Center Groningen, University of Groningen, 9713 GZ Groningen, The Netherlands
* Correspondence: f.f.a.ijpma@umcg.nl; Tel.: +31-503616161
† This work was presented in part as A.M.L. Meesters's Ph.D. Thesis at the University of Groningen (2022).

Abstract: This study aims to develop a three-dimensional (3D) measurement for acetabular fracture displacement, determine the inter- and intra-observer variability, and correlate the measurement with clinical outcome. Three-dimensional models were created for 100 patients surgically treated for acetabular fractures. The '3D gap area', the 3D surface between all the fracture fragments, was developed. The association between the 3D gap area and the risk of conversion to a total hip arthroplasty (THA) was determined by an ROC curve and a Cox regression analysis. The 3D gap area had an excellent inter-observer and intra-observer reliability. The preoperative median 3D gap area for patients without and with a THA was 1731 mm^2 versus 2237 mm^2. The median postoperative 3D gap area was 640 mm^2 versus 845 mm^2. The area under the curve was 0.63. The Cox regression analysis showed that a preoperative 3D gap area > 2103 mm^2 and a postoperative 3D gap area > 1058 mm^2 were independently associated with a 3.0 versus 2.4 times higher risk of conversion to a THA. A 3D assessment of acetabular fractures is feasible, reproducible, and correlates with clinical outcome. Three-dimensional measurements could be added to the current classification systems to quantify the level of fracture displacement and to assess operative results.

Keywords: acetabular fracture; 3D fracture analysis; 3D gap area; three dimensional; three-dimensional measurements; 3DCT

1. Introduction

The incidence of acetabular fractures, i.e., fractures involving the hip socket, is estimated as 5 to 8 per 100,000 people per year [1,2]. These fractures can have a serious influence on physical functioning, social activities, and the ability to work. In general, minimally displaced fractures can be treated nonoperatively, and this accounts for approximately half of all acetabular fractures [3,4]. Displaced fractures are mostly treated surgically with reduction and internal fixation; only a small percentage of patients need a primary total hip arthroplasty (THA) [3,5]. The main goal of surgical treatment is to obtain an accurate reconstruction of the articular surface in order to minimize the risk of progressive osteoarthritis and the subsequent need for a THA [6,7]. The residual fracture displacement, measured as the two-dimensional (2D) gap and step-off on computed tomography (CT) slices, is an important factor for estimating the risk for conversion to a THA after surgical treatment of an acetabular fracture. Verbeek et al. reported that an anatomical reduction, according to Matta's criteria [8] (0–1 mm residual displacement), leads to only 3 percent

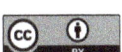

conversion to a THA, whereas poor reduction (>3 mm residual displacement) leads to 36 percent conversion to a THA after acetabular fractures after a mean follow-up of nine years [9]. They measured the postoperative reduction on radiographs and 2DCT slices. However, these 2D gap and step-off measurements of the initial fracture displacement and postoperative fracture reduction suffer from low inter- and intra-observer agreement [10]. If surgeons still cannot fully agree on the degree of fracture displacement, it will be difficult to assess the results of acetabular fracture surgery and estimate the prognosis by using conventional 2D measurements techniques.

Acetabular fractures usually consist of multiple fracture fragments, which can be displaced in multiple dimensions. The current AO/OTA (Arbeitsgemeinschaft für Osteosynthesefragen/Orthopaedic Trauma Association) classification system only describes the gross fracture pattern but does not include information about the degree of displacement of each fracture fragment [11]. Obtaining insights into the extent of the fracture displacement can be difficult using only 2DCT slices [12]. An understanding of the complexity of the fracture is necessary for determining the treatment strategy, providing the best possible surgical treatment, evaluating the postoperative result, and estimating the prognosis [13]. Three-dimensional imaging and measurements can provide insight into the multidirectional displacement of the fracture fragments and can quantify the true extent of the fracture displacement [14–17]. Recently, we introduced a 3DCT measurement method for acetabular fractures and compared these measurements with the gold standard 2D gap and step-off measurements [18]. The 3DCT reduction criteria were suggested in previous research [18], but these consist of multiple items, including the 3D gap, 3D step-off, and the total gap area (a 2D surface measurement on a 3D fracture model). Because it is unknown which item is the most important, it can be complicated to decide which criteria must be used in clinical practice and differences between users may occur. Thus, no universal measurement exists that incorporates both the gaps and step-offs between multiple fracture fragments into one measurement. Moreover, the currently available 3DCT measurement method has not been correlated with clinical outcome.

The study did not aim to evaluate the quality of the surgery, but the aim was to test the feasibility of a newly developed measurement method. We hypothesize that a single 3DCT measurement for acetabular fractures will provide an observer-independent analysis of the complexity of the fracture and can be one of the factors that indicate whether a patient is at risk for a THA during follow-up. The aim was to validate our developed 3D measurement method by answering the following research questions: (1) What is the inter- and intra-observer variability of a single 3DCT measurement for the initial and residual displacement in surgically treated acetabular fractures? (2) Is there a relationship between the preoperative 3D measurement and the risk of conversion to a total hip arthroplasty during follow-up? (3) Is there a relationship between the postoperative 3D measurement and the risk of conversion to a total hip arthroplasty in follow-up?

2. Materials and Methods

2.1. Patients

A diagnostic imaging study was performed in patients treated for acetabular fractures in a level 1 trauma center. Between 2001 and 2020, we treated 428 patients for an acetabular fracture. Of those, we considered surgically treated unilateral acetabular fractures with availability of a high-quality pre- and postoperative CT-scan (with a maximum slice thickness of 2 mm and acquired within four weeks after surgery) and at least one-year clinical follow-up as potentially eligible. Based on that, 63% (270) were eligible; a further 10% (42) were excluded because they were treated with a primary THA (6), were under 18 years old (6), had a periprosthetic fracture (3), had a concomitant pelvic ring injury (24) or a pipkin femoral head fracture (3), and another 30% (128) were deceased (23), were lost prior to the minimum study follow-up of one year (17), or had incomplete datasets (18 patients missing a preoperative CT scan, 45 patients missing a postoperative CT scan, and 25 patients with poor quality CT scans with a slice thickness larger than 2 mm), thus leaving 23% (100) for analysis here. Baseline characteristics were retrieved from the patients' medical records. All pelvic CT scans at the time of injury were reassessed by two trauma surgeons (KtD, FIJ) and all fractures were classified according to the Letournel classification [19]. All available fracture types were included to prevent potential bias. In our clinic, pre- and postoperative CT scans became standard of care over the past seven years. Before that time, the CT scans were performed based on surgeons' preferences or indication. Patients were approached by telephone or posted mail and asked whether they received a THA after their acetabular fracture surgery. Indications for conversion to THA were progressive symptomatic osteoarthritis (24/31, Kellgren–Lawrence grade 4 [20]) and avascular necrosis of the femoral head (7/31). Moreover, follow-up information regarding THA was retrieved from the patients' medical records.

This study was reviewed, and a waiver was provided by the Medical Ethics Review Committee of the University Medical Center Groningen, no: 2016.385. This study is reported following Strengthening the Reporting of Observational Studies in Epidemiology (STROBE) reporting guideline.

2.2. Three-Dimensional Measurements

Three-dimensional models were created based on the pre- and postoperative CT scans, using the segmentation-certified software of Mimics Medical software (version 19.0; Materialise, Leuven, Belgium). A preset threshold for bone ($\geq$226 Hounsfield Units) was used and all the different fracture fragments were manually separated into individual 3D objects. All 3D objects were imported into the certified 3-matic Medical software (version 13.0; Materialise, Leuven, Belgium). The measurements were first performed on the 3D models derived from the preoperative CT scans. The surface along the edge of the fracture fragments (e.g., the fracture line) was marked (Figure 1a) and separated from the 3D model. The contours of this surface were converted to curves. These curves were trimmed so that the line that remained solely covered the fragments' fracture edge (Figure 1b). The fracture lines were connected so one enclosed curve was created, which resembled the border of the 3D gap area (Figure 1c). Based on this closed curve, a surface was generated using the surface construction function in 3-matic (Figure 1d). This final generated surface, so called 3D gap area, represents the fracture area (mm^2) between all fracture fragments. To measure the postoperative 3D gap area, the preoperative fracture fragments were matched with the postoperative 3D model using surface-based matching to avoid the possible influence of metal artefacts. The corresponding preoperative fracture lines were translated together with the fracture fragments and used to determine the 3D gap area postoperatively. All pre- and postoperative 3D models were measured by one observer (AM) experienced in using the 3D software, and it takes on average about two hours per patient to create the 3D models and measure the 3D gap area. Two-dimensional measurements were not included in this study, because previous research showed unreliable results for these measurements [10,18,21].

2.3. Statistical Analysis

To answer our first question, regarding the inter- and intra-observer variability of a single 3DCT measurement, twenty pre- and postoperative 3D models were measured by two additional experienced observers (MO, NA). The intraclass correlation coefficient (ICC), with a two-way mixed, single measurements model with absolute agreement, and the 95% confidence interval (CI) were calculated using SPSS (version 23, IBM, Chicago, IL, USA). Moreover, the median difference and interquartile range (IQR) between the values measured by the different observers were calculated. Finally, one observer (AM) repeated all the twenty measurements two times, with an interval of at least one week, and the ICC with 95% CI were calculated to investigate the intra-observer variability.

To answer the second and third question, regarding the relationship between the 3D measurement and the risk of conversion to total hip arthroplasty, the median and IQR were calculated for all continuous data. Frequencies and percentages were calculated for all dichotomous data. The median pre- and postoperative 3D gap area was calculated for all patients. Next, the median pre- and postoperative 3D gap area was calculated for the group of patients with a THA and for the group of patients that retained their native hip. The Mann–Whitney U test was used to compare groups. Finally, a receiver operating characteristics (ROC) curve was created to assess whether the 3D gap area and conversion to THA were related. Critical cut-off values for the pre- as well as postoperative 3D gap area, based on the increased risk of THA, were determined by the value for which the combined sensitivity and specificity is the highest (Youden's J statistic). These cut-off values were used in a Cox regression analysis for assessing the association between 3D gap area and the risk of conversion to THA and determining a hazard ratio (HR).

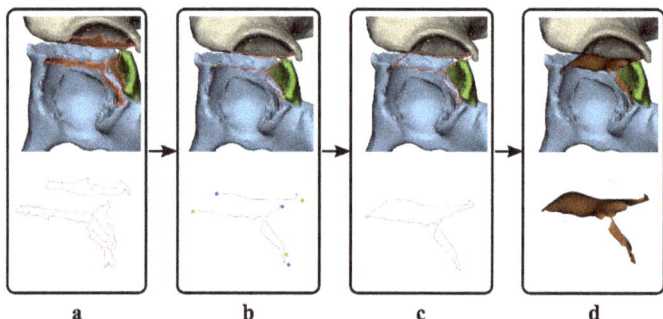

Figure 1. Method for determining the three-dimensional (3D) gap area. (**a**) The surface on the edge of each fracture fragment (e.g., fracture line) is marked (top) and the contours of the surface are converted to curves (red, bottom). (**b**) The curves are cut so that only the fracture lines remain. (**c**) The fracture lines are connected to generate an enclosed curve. (**d**) A three-dimensional surface, the 3D gap area, is generated based on the closed curve of the fracture lines (orange).

3. Results

3.1. Patients

The median (IQR) age of the included patients was 49 (38–63) years (Table 1). Twenty-eight out of a hundred patients received a THA after a median (IQR) of 16 (11–27) months. Additionally, three patients had an indication for a THA due to symptomatic osteoarthritis (Kellgren–Lawrence grade 4 on follow-up radiograph [20]). They did not receive a THA, because the patients chose to refrain from revision surgery due to comorbidities. These patients were analyzed in the THA group.

Table 1. Patient characteristics. THA: Total hip arthroplasty.

Patient Demographics (N = 100)			
	Native Hip (N = 69)	THA (N = 31)	Total
Sex (no.)			
Male	59	24	83
Female	10	7	17
Median (IQR) age (in years)	48 (34–62)	53 (41–67)	49 (38–64)
Letournel classification (no.)			
Anterior column	5	1	6
Posterior column	1	0	1
Posterior wall	15	6	21
Transverse	1	0	1
Anterior column and posterior hemitransverse	6	0	6
Both column	23	9	32
Posterior column and posterior wall	4	3	7
T-type	8	3	11
Transverse and posterior wall	6	9	15

3.2. Inter- and Intra-Observer Reliability

The inter- and intra-observer reliability was excellent for the pre- and postoperative 3D gap area. For the inter-observer measurements of the 3D gap area, the preoperative ICC was 0.95 (95% CI: 0.84–0.98) and the postoperative ICC was 0.95 (95% CI: 0.89–0.98). The median difference (IQR) between the observers was 182 (102–260) mm^2 preoperatively and 174 (91–283) mm^2 postoperatively. For the intra-observer measurements, the preoperative ICC was 0.96 (95% CI: 0.91–0.98) and the postoperative ICC was 0.99 (95% CI: 0.97–0.99). The median difference (IQR) between the repeated measurements was 83 (40–124) mm^2 preoperatively and 58 (33–115) mm^2 postoperatively.

3.3. Preoperative 3D Measurement Correlated with Clinical Outcome

The preoperative 3D gap area is associated with clinical outcome. The overall median (IQR) preoperative 3D gap area for all 100 patients was 1867 (1261–2411) mm^2. For patients who retained their native hip (N = 69), the median (IQR) preoperative 3D gap area was 1731 (1075–2446) mm^2 compared to 2237 (1775–2393) mm^2 (p = 0.045) for patients in the THA group (N = 31). The area under the curve was 0.63 (95% CI: 0.51–0.74, p = 0.045) for the preoperative 3D gap area (Figure 2). The preoperative critical cut-off value for a conversion to a THA was 2103 mm^2 with a sensitivity of 61% and a specificity of 73%. The Cox regression analysis, adjusted for age and gender, showed that a preoperative 3D gap area > 2103 mm^2 (critical cut-off) was independently associated with a 3.0 times higher risk of conversion to a THA (adjusted: HR 3.0, 95% CI: 1.4–6.2, p = 0.004; unadjusted: HR 3.1, 95% CI: 1.5–6.4, p = 0.002).

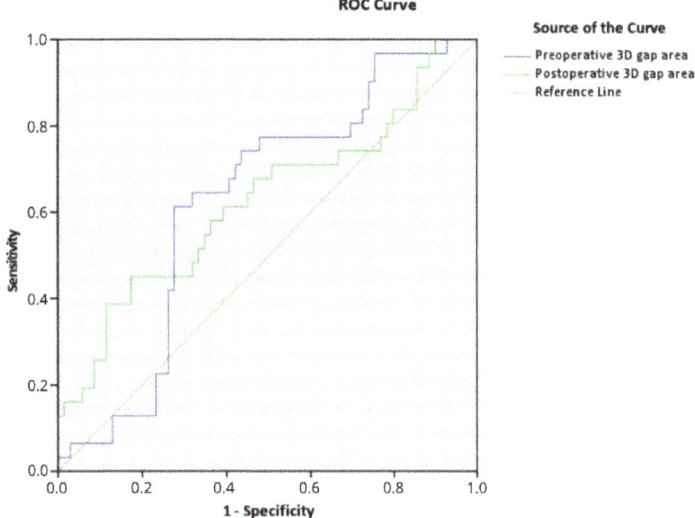

Figure 2. Receiver operating characteristic (ROC) curve demonstrating that the pre- and postoperative 3D gap area are associated with conversion to total hip arthroplasty.

3.4. Postoperative 3D Measurement Correlated with Clinical Outcome

The postoperative 3D gap area is associated with clinical outcome. The overall median (IQR) postoperative 3D gap area for all 100 patients was 679 (310–1074) mm^2. The median (IQR) postoperative 3D gap area was 640 (311–961) mm^2 for patients who retained their native hip, compared to 845 (298–1456) mm^2 for patients in the THA group (p = 0.045). For the postoperative 3D gap area, the area under the curve was 0.63 (95% CI: 0.50–0.75, p = 0.045). The postoperative critical cut-off value was 1058 mm^2 with a sensitivity of 45% and a specificity of 83% for a conversion to a THA. The Cox regression analysis, adjusted for age and gender, showed that a postoperative 3D gap area > 1058 mm^2 (critical cut-off) was independently associated with a 2.4 times higher risk of conversion to a THA (adjusted: HR 2.4, 95% CI: 1.1–5.2, p = 0.021; unadjusted: HR 2.7, 95% CI: 1.3–5.5, p = 0.006). The clinical case examples of the 3D gap area are shown in Figures 3, 4, S1 and S2.

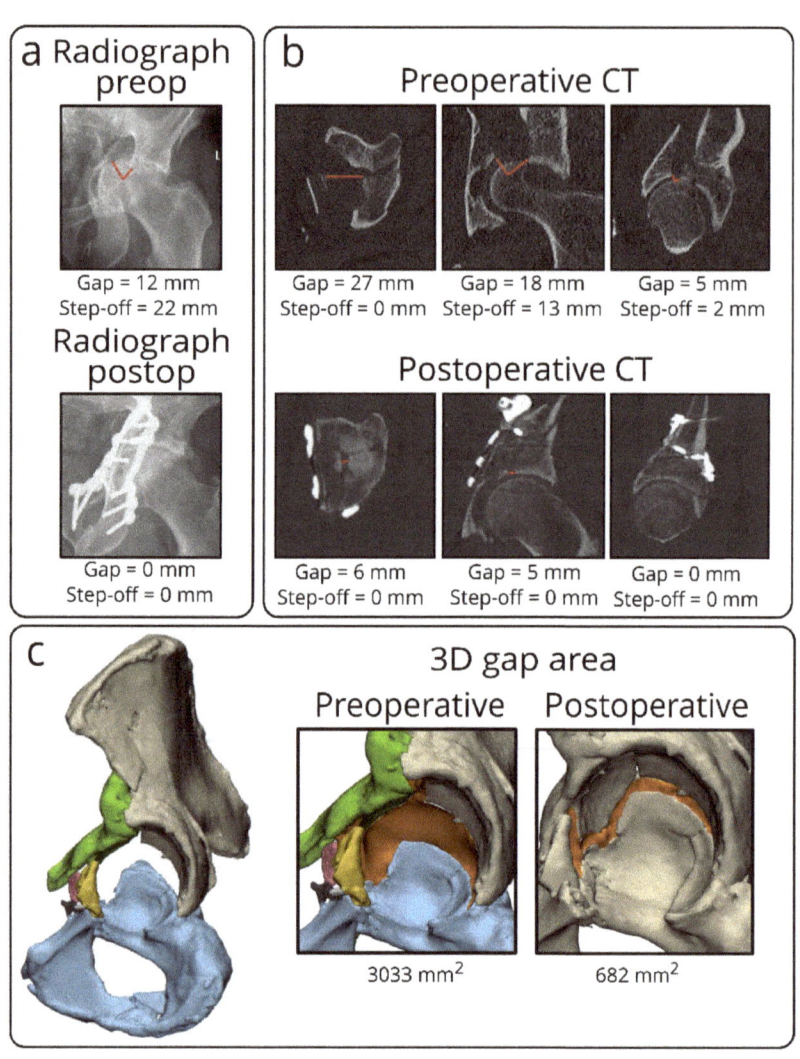

Figure 3. Case example of a both-column fracture in a 63-year-old male, showing the discrepancy in measuring initial and residual fracture displacement for acetabular fractures on different imaging modalities, including radiographs, CT scans, and 3D models. On radiographs (**a**), it is difficult to measure gaps and step-offs, especially on the postoperative radiograph, because the implant is partially obscuring the acetabulum. On the single CT slices (**b**), multiple gaps and step-offs (red lines) can be measured on different CT slices in several planes, indicating the subjective elements of these measurements. The 3D model (**c**) demonstrates the 3D gap area (in orange) representing the three-dimensional surface between all fracture fragments. This should be considered a single quantitative measure of the initial or residual fracture displacement in the entire acetabulum.

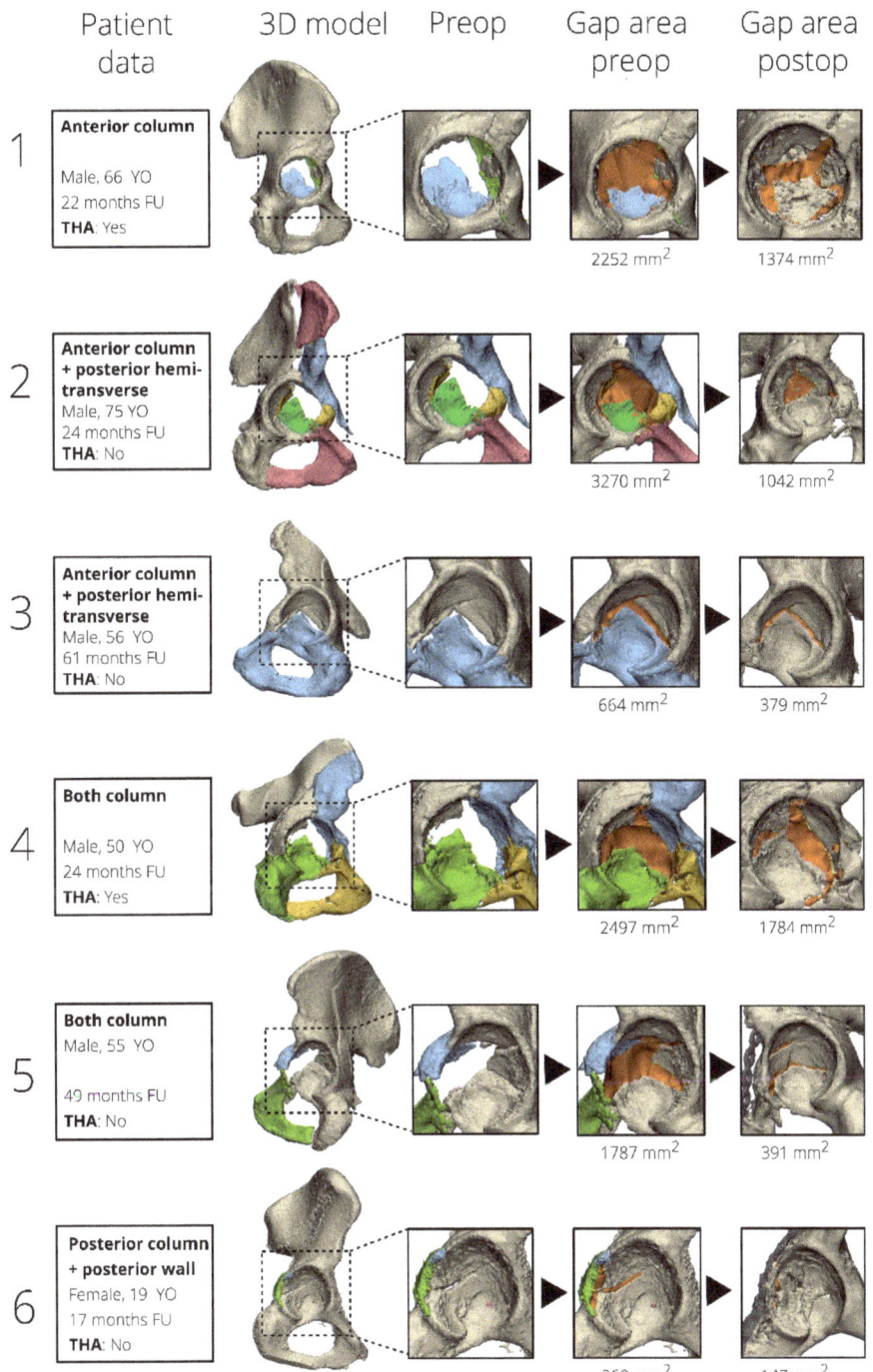

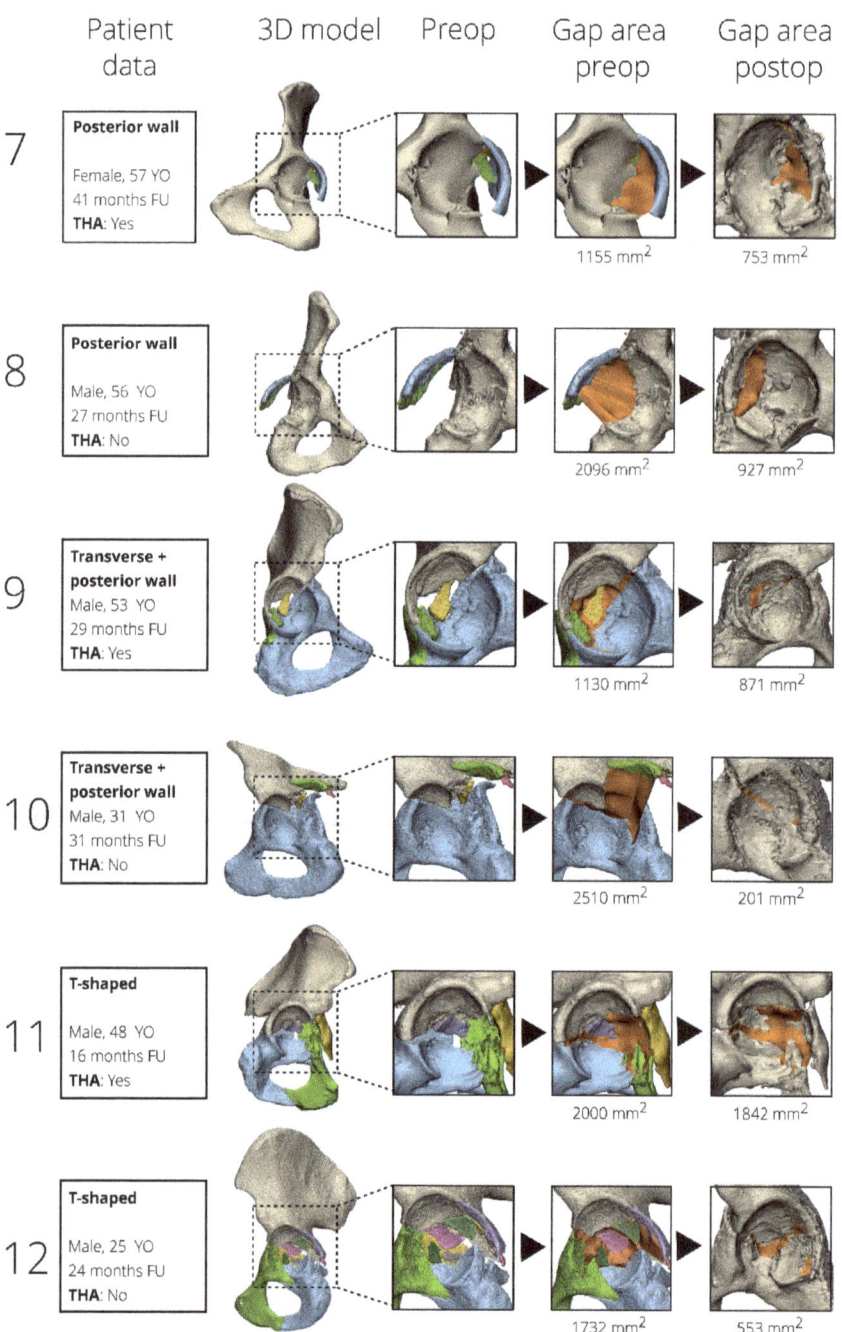

Figure 4. Case examples of 12 patients, surgically treated for different types of acetabular fractures, are presented in order to correlate fracture displacement (as measured by the 3D gap area, orange) to clinical outcome. The pre- and postoperative 3D gap area are indicated in orange. The cases are sorted based on fracture type. YO: years old, FU: follow-up, THA: total hip arthroplasty.

4. Discussion

The conventional 2DCT single slice gap and step-off measurements of an initial fracture displacement and postoperative fracture reduction, which are currently used to evaluate the results of acetabular fracture surgery, suffer from low inter- and intra-observer agreement and do not represent the displacement of all fracture fragments [10]. The aim of this study was to develop and evaluate our single 3DCT measurement in order to quantify the preoperative fracture displacement and postoperative reduction in acetabular fracture surgery by determining the inter- and intra-observer variability and investigating the relationship between the 3D measurement and the risk of conversion to a THA. We introduced the 3D gap area measurement that represents the 3D surface area between all fracture fragments. The measure was developed and assessed on the pre- and postoperative 3D models of 100 patients. Our study shows that the 3D gap area can be reliably measured and accurately reproduced, with high inter- and intra-observer reliability. The 3D gap area measurements represent an observer-independent single quantitative measure for assessing the initial fracture displacement and postoperative fracture reduction. Patients who needed a THA had a higher median pre- and postoperative 3D gap area compared to those who retained their native hip, indicating that the 3D gap area is associated with clinical outcome.

This study contains several limitations. First of all, the 3D software, 3D expertise, and manpower needed for the measurements are not available in all hospitals. Second, there is a selection bias, because only the patients with a postoperative CT scan were included. These postoperative CT scans were only made standard of care over the last 7 years, whereas before this time, a postoperative CT scan was only performed upon indication. However, this does not affect our research method, because our study aimed to introduce and assess a 3D measurement technique and link those to the risk of conversion to a THA instead of reporting on the clinical outcome itself. Finally, creating 3D models and performing the 3D gap area measurements is time-consuming and will take on average two hours per patient. Yet, future developments in software might reduce this time, making it more applicable in clinical practice.

Accuracy and reproducibility of measurements for assessing fracture displacement is mandatory to use them with confidence in clinical practice. In this study, we introduced a new 3D measurement for assessing acetabular fracture displacement that is accurate, reliable, and does not depend on the subjective interpretations of surgeons. The gap and step-off measurements using traditional 2D imaging (e.g., radiographs or 2DCT slices) have proven to be insufficient for assessing the displacement of acetabular fractures [10,21]. The assessment of a fracture relies on where the 2D measurement is performed, meaning which fracture line or CT slice is selected for the measurement and how the measurement is performed. A previous study demonstrated a low inter-observer reliability of the gap and step-off measurements on 2DCT slices, with ICCs varying from 0.3–0.4 [10]. The unique feature of our new 3D gap area measurement is that it includes the entire fractured area and combines the gaps and step-offs between all fracture fragments in one 3D surface. This approach enables expressing the degree of initial and residual fracture displacement in a single quantitative measure for the first time.

Quantifying the initial fracture displacement and postoperative reduction is essential for the treatment decision and patient counseling regarding the prognosis. The 3D gap area was correlated with conversion to a THA in order to assess whether it could potentially be used as a predictive value for the clinical outcome. The median initial displacement (preoperative 3D gap area) and the median residual displacement (postoperative 3D gap area) were higher in the group of patients that received a THA during follow-up, indicating that the 3D gap area is associated with clinical outcome. Moreover, if the preoperative 3D gap area can be used to predict the risk of conversion to a THA during follow-up, this could have major implications in deciding about osteosynthesis versus a primary THA at the time of the injury. This study provides a preliminary critical cut-off value for the preoperative 3D gap area (>2103 mm^2; HR 3.0, 95% CI 1.4–6.2; $p = 0.004$), which is independently associated with the risk of conversion to a THA. Obviously, definitive cut-off values for relating the

3D gap area to the risk of conversion to a THA still need to be determined in a larger series. On the other hand, we noticed that the pre- and postoperative 3D gap area does not always correlate with clinical outcome. For instance, one patient with a relatively small pre- and postoperative 3D gap area (625 and 205 mm^2, e.g., indicating limited initial displacement and proper fracture reduction) eventually received a THA due to avascular necrosis of the femoral head instead of due to progressive osteoarthritis caused by residual fracture displacement. In this study, pre- and postoperative 3D gap areas still have moderate discriminating ability (area under the curve of 0.63) between whether or not a conversion to a THA will be needed at follow-up. This might be explained by the fact that multiple patient factors, including age, comorbidity, femoral head injuries, and dome impaction, are associated with clinical outcome as well. Another important parameter could be the location of the fracture displacement, e.g., a fracture of the weightbearing dome might be more likely to cause osteoarthritis and conversion to a THA. A larger multicenter follow-up study, including both patient as well as fracture characteristics, is needed to unravel the true discriminating ability of the 3D gap area. Overall, the introduction of our 3D gap area for assessing the fracture displacement should be considered as a first step away from the traditional observer-dependent 2D gap and step-off measurements and toward a new era of a standardized advanced 3D evaluation of operative results. The 3D technology for acetabular fracture surgery has been increasingly used around the world in the past few years [22]. We envision that an automatic segmentation and (semi-)automated 3D analysis of fracture displacement will be possible in the near future. For instance, the 3D gap area measurement could be integrated in commercially available surgical planning software in order to standardize the evaluations of the operation results and eventually estimate prognosis.

The 3D gap area measurement represents a reproducible single measurement to quantify the initial fracture displacement and postoperative fracture reduction in acetabular fracture treatment. The unique aspect of this measurement is that it includes the entire fractured area and incorporates gaps and step-offs between all fracture fragments in one 3D surface. Moreover, it is a single quantitative measure that is associated with clinical outcome. In general, we envision that 3D measurements of fracture displacement will open a new era of evaluating operation results.

Supplementary Materials: The following supporting information can be downloaded at: https://www.mdpi.com/article/10.3390/jpm12091464/s1, **Figure S1:** Pre- and postoperative 3D gap area. Three-dimensional gap area measurement (indicated in orange) showing the preoperative (initial) and postoperative (residual) fracture displacement of a 39-year-old woman with a transverse-posterior wall type of acetabular fracture. The preoperative 3D gap area was 1251 mm^2 and the postoperative 3D gap area was 324 mm^2. **Figure S2:** Both-column examples. Case examples of four patients, surgically treated for both-column acetabular fractures, are presented in order to visually correlate fracture displacement (as measured by the 3D gap area) to clinical and radiological outcome. The pre- and postoperative 3D gap area is indicated in orange. Patients who had conversion to THA at follow-up had osteoarthritis on the follow-up radiograph. YO: years old, FU: follow-up, THA: total hip arthroplasty.

Author Contributions: Conceptualization, A.M.L.M., N.A., J.K. and F.F.A.I.; methodology, A.M.L.M., N.A., J.K. and F.F.A.I.; software, A.M.L.M., M.G.E.O. and N.A.; validation, A.M.L.M., M.G.E.O., N.M.T., N.A., J.K., M.J.H.W., J.-P.P.M.d.V., K.t.D. and F.F.A.I.; formal analysis, A.M.L.M., M.G.E.O., N.M.T., N.A., J.K., M.J.H.W., J.-P.P.M.d.V., K.t.D. and F.F.A.I.; investigation, A.M.L.M., M.G.E.O., N.A. and F.F.A.I.; resources, A.M.L.M. and N.M.T.; data curation, A.M.L.M. and M.G.E.O.; writing—original draft preparation, A.M.L.M., M.G.E.O., N.A. and F.F.A.I.; writing—review and editing, N.M.T., J.K., M.J.H.W., J.-P.P.M.d.V. and K.t.D.; visualization, A.M.L.M. and M.G.E.O.; supervision, J.K., M.J.H.W., J.-P.P.M.d.V., K.t.D. and F.F.A.I.; project administration, A.M.L.M.; funding acquisition, not applicable. All authors have read and agreed to the published version of the manuscript.

Funding: This research received no external funding.

Institutional Review Board Statement: Ethical review and approval were waived for this study due to treatment according to standard of care and patients were only once contacted.

Informed Consent Statement: Patient consent was waived due to treatment according to standard of care and patients were only once contacted.

Data Availability Statement: The authors declare that the data supporting the findings of this study are available within the paper.

Acknowledgments: We would like to thank Hester Banierink, for helping to gather patient data.

Conflicts of Interest: The authors declare no conflict of interest.

References

1. Rinne, P.P.; Laitinen, M.K.; Huttunen, T.; Kannus, P.; Mattila, V.M. The incidence and trauma mechanisms of acetabular fractures: A nationwide study in Finland between 1997 and 2014. *Injury* **2017**, *48*, 2157–2161. [CrossRef] [PubMed]
2. Melhem, E.; Riouallon, G.; Habboubi, K.; Gabbas, M.; Jouffroy, P. Epidemiology of pelvic and acetabular fractures in France. *Orthop. Traumatol. Surg. Res.* **2020**, *106*, 831–839. [CrossRef] [PubMed]
3. Boudissa, M.; Francony, F.; Kerschbaumer, G.; Ruatti, S.; Milaire, M.; Merloz, P.; Tonetti, J. Epidemiology and treatment of acetabular fractures in a level-1 trauma centre: Retrospective study of 414 patients over 10 years. *Orthop. Traumatol. Surg. Res.* **2017**, *103*, 335–339. [CrossRef] [PubMed]
4. Clarke-Jenssen, J.; Wikerøy, A.K.; Røise, O.; Øvre, S.A.; Madsen, J.E. Long-term survival of the native hip after a minimally displaced, nonoperatively treated acetabular fracture. *J. Bone Jt. Surg. Am.* **2016**, *98*, 1392–1399. [CrossRef]
5. Grubor, P.; Krupic, F.; Biscevic, M.; Grubor, M. Controversies in treatment of acetabular fracture. *Med. Arch. (Sarajevo, Bosnia Herzegovina)* **2015**, *69*, 16–20. [CrossRef]
6. Verbeek, D.O.; van der List, J.P.; Tissue, C.M.; Helfet, D.L. Long-term patient reported outcomes following acetabular fracture fixation. *Injury* **2018**, *49*, 1131–1136. [CrossRef]
7. Giannoudis, P.V.; Grotz, M.R.W.; Papakostidis, C.; Dinopoulos, H. Operative treatment of displaced fractures of the acetabulum. A meta-analysis. *J. Bone Jt. Surgery. Br. Vol.* **2005**, *87*, 2–9. [CrossRef]
8. Matta, J.M. Fractures of the acetabulum: Accuracy of reduction and clinical results in patients managed operatively within three weeks after the injury. *J. Bone Joint Surg. Am.* **1996**, *78*, 1632–1645. [CrossRef]
9. Verbeek, D.O.; Van Der List, J.P.; Villa, J.C.; Wellman, D.S.; Helfet, D.L. Postoperative CT is superior for acetabular fracture reduction assessment and reliably predicts hip survivorship. *J. Bone Jt. Surg. Am. Vol.* **2017**, *99*, 1745–1752. [CrossRef]
10. Meesters, A.M.L.; ten Duis, K.; Banierink, H.; Stirler, V.M.A.; Wouters, P.C.R.; Kraeima, J.; De Vries, J.-P.P.M.; Witjes, M.J.H.; Ijpma, F.F.A. What are the interobserver and intraobserver variability of gap and stepoff measurements in acetabular fractures? *Clin. Orthop. Relat. Res.* **2020**, *478*, 2801–2808. [CrossRef]
11. Meinberg, E.G.; Agel, J.; Roberts, C.S.; Karam, M.D.; Kellam, J.F. Fracture and dislocation classification compendium—2018. *J. Orthop. Trauma* **2018**, *32*, S1–S10. [CrossRef] [PubMed]
12. Scheinfeld, M.H.; Dym, A.A.; Spektor, M.; Avery, L.L.; Dym, R.J.; Amanatullah, D.F. Acetabular fractures: What radiologists should know and how 3D CT can aid classification. *RadioGraphics* **2015**, *35*, 555–577. [CrossRef] [PubMed]
13. Matta, J.M. Operative indications and choice of surgical approach for fractures of the acetabulum. *Technol. Orthop.* **1986**, *1*, 13–22. [CrossRef]
14. Mellema, J.J.; Janssen, S.J.; Guitton, T.; Ring, D. Quantitative 3-dimensional computed tomography measurements of coronoid fractures. *J. Hand Surg.* **2015**, *40*, 526–533. [CrossRef]
15. Lubberts, B.; Janssen, S.; Mellema, J.; Ring, D. Quantitative 3-dimensional computed tomography analysis of olecranon fractures. *J. Shoulder Elb. Surg.* **2015**, *25*, 831–836. [CrossRef]
16. De Muinck Keizer, R.-J.O.; Meijer, D.T.; van der Gronde, B.A.T.D.; Teunis, T.; Stufkens, S.A.S.; Kerkhoffs, G.M.; Goslings, J.C.; Doornberg, J.N. Articular gap and step-off revisited: 3D quantification of operative reduction for posterior malleolar fragments. *J. Orthop. Trauma* **2016**, *30*, 670–675. [CrossRef]
17. Assink, N.; Kraeima, J.; Slump, C.H.; Duis, K.T.; De Vries, J.P.P.M.; Meesters, A.M.L.; van Ooijen, P.; Witjes, M.; Ijpma, F.F.A. Quantitative 3D measurements of tibial plateau fractures. *Sci. Rep.* **2019**, *9*, 14395. [CrossRef]
18. Meesters, A.M.L.; Kraeima, J.; Banierink, H.; Slump, C.H.; De Vries, J.P.P.M.; ten Duis, K.; Witjes, M.J.H.; Ijpma, F.F.A. Introduction of a three-dimensional computed tomography measurement method for acetabular fractures. *PLoS ONE* **2019**, *14*, e0218612. [CrossRef]
19. Tile, M.; Helfet, D.L.; Kellam, J.F.; Vrahas, M. *Fractures of the Pelvis and Acetabulum—Principles and Methods of Management*, 4th ed.; Georg Thieme Verlag: Stuttgart, Germany; New York, NY, USA, 2015; ISBN 9781604062090.
20. Kellgren, J.; Lawrence, J. Radiological assessment of osteo-arthrosis. *Ann. Rheum. Dis.* **1957**, *16*, 494–502. [CrossRef]

21. Meesters, A.M.L.; ten Duis, K.; Kraeima, J.; Banierink, H.; Stirler, V.M.A.; Wouters, P.C.R.; de Vries, J.P.P.M.; Witjes, M.J.H.; IJpma, F.F.A. The accuracy of gap and step-off measurements in acetabular fracture treatment. *Sci. Rep.* **2021**, *11*, 18294. [CrossRef]
22. Meesters, A.M.L.; Trouwborst, N.M.; De Vries, J.P.M.; Kraeima, J.; Witjes, M.J.H.; Doornberg, J.N.; Reininga, I.H.F.; IJpma, F.F.A.; ten Duis, K. Does 3D-Assisted Acetabular Fracture Surgery Improve Surgical Outcome and Physical Functioning ?— A Systematic Review. *J. Pers. Med.* **2021**, *11*, 966. [CrossRef] [PubMed]

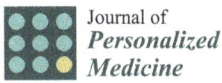

Article

Four-Dimensional Determination of the Patient-Specific Centre of Rotation for Total Temporomandibular Joint Replacements: Following the Groningen Principle

Bram B. J. Merema *, Max J. H. Witjes, Nicolaas B. Van Bakelen, Joep Kraeima and Frederik K. L. Spijkervet

Department of Oral and Maxillofacial Surgery, University Medical Center Groningen, University of Groningen, Hanzeplein 1, P.O. Box 30.001, 9700 RB Groningen, The Netherlands
* Correspondence: b.j.merema@umcg.nl; Tel.: +31 503610213

Abstract: For patients who suffer from severe dysfunction of the temporomandibular joint (TMJ), a total joint replacement (TJR) in the form of a prosthesis may be indicated. The position of the centre of rotation in TJRs is crucial for good postoperative oral function; however, it is not determined patient-specifically (PS) in any current TMJ-TJR. The aim of this current study was to develop a 4D-workflow to ascertain the PS mean axis of rotation, or fixed hinge, that mimics the patient's specific physiological mouth opening. Twenty healthy adult patients were asked to volunteer for a 4D-scanning procedure. From these 4D-scanning recordings of mouth opening exercises, patient-specific centres of rotation and axes of rotation were determined using our JawAnalyser tool. The mean CR location was positioned 28 [mm] inferiorly and 5.5 [mm] posteriorly to the centre of condyle (CoC). The 95% confidence interval ranged from 22.9 to 33.7 [mm] inferior and 3.1 to 7.8 [mm] posterior to the CoC. This study succeeded in developing an accurate 4D-workflow to determine a PS mean axis of rotation that mimics the patient's specific physiological mouth opening. Furthermore, a change in concept is necessary for all commercially available TMJ-TJR prostheses in order to comply with the PS CRs calculated by our study. In the meantime, it seems wise to stick to placing the CR 15 [mm] inferiorly to the CoC, or even beyond, towards 28 [mm] if the patient's anatomy allows this.

Keywords: mandible; jaw; 4D; motion analysis; kinematic; patient-specific; custom; prosthesis; TMJ; TJR; 3D-VSP; virtual surgical planning

Citation: Merema, B.B.J.; Witjes, M.J.H.; Van Bakelen, N.B.; Kraeima, J.; Spijkervet, F.K.L. Four-Dimensional Determination of the Patient-Specific Centre of Rotation for Total Temporomandibular Joint Replacements: Following the Groningen Principle. *J. Pers. Med.* **2022**, *12*, 1439. https://doi.org/10.3390/jpm12091439

Academic Editor: Jung-Wook Kim

Received: 10 August 2022
Accepted: 26 August 2022
Published: 31 August 2022

Publisher's Note: MDPI stays neutral with regard to jurisdictional claims in published maps and institutional affiliations.

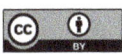

Copyright: © 2022 by the authors. Licensee MDPI, Basel, Switzerland. This article is an open access article distributed under the terms and conditions of the Creative Commons Attribution (CC BY) license (https://creativecommons.org/licenses/by/4.0/).

1. Introduction

A total joint replacement (TJR) of the temporomandibular joint (TMJ) in the form of a prosthesis may be indicated for patients who suffer from severe TMJ dysfunction. Documented indications include end-stage degenerative joint disease, recurrent ankylosis, and congenital disorders affecting the TMJ when joint saving approaches do not suffice [1]. Other indications for TJRs are condylar loss as a result of trauma or neoplasia in or near the joint or to replace a failed alloplastic or autogenous reconstruction [2]. In most of these patients, mandibular movement is impaired due to either anatomical changes or surgically caused scarification, often resulting in pain, difficulties in speech, impaired oral function, and limited maximum mouth opening.

When replacing the TMJ with a TMJ-TJR prosthesis, the condyle or its remnants together with the articular disc are removed in order to fit the prosthesis. This results in the removal of the insertion of the main muscle responsible for anterior movement of the condyle, the lateral pterygoid muscle, from its insertions at the mandibular condyle and articular disc. Removal of this muscle's insertion site in order to place a TMJ-TJR is reported to decrease the amount of anterior movement of the TMJ from approximately 16 [mm] to only 2 [mm] [3] or less, thereby reducing the joint's movements to near mere rotations [4]. The consequences of placing a TMJ-TJR unilaterally are a lack of anterior movement leading to asymmetrical mouth opening movements, where the mandible deviates towards the affected side, marginal laterotrusion towards the unaffected side [5], and unnatural loading of the contralateral joint [6].

To overcome this effect, the Groningen TMJ-TJR prosthesis was developed [7–9]. Apart from its unique feature that allows for free translational movement of the neo-disc, the prosthesis applies a lowered centre of rotation (CR) in relation to the anatomical condylar centre [8]. Prior research suggested that a lowering of 15 [mm] in relation to the condyle would be optimal as a fixed CR for unilateral TMJ prostheses [3]. This study was, however, based on 2D optical movement tracking with no direct relation to the bony anatomy and thus the condyles of the mandible [10]. The Groningen TMJ-TJR prosthesis has been available as a patient-specific (PS) device since 2017, opening doors to also personalise the position of the CR [8]. Figure 1 illustrates the effect of a lowered centre of rotation with the Groningen TMJ-TJR prosthesis.

Physiological mandibular movement is complex and, as per definition, not truly translatable to a mere rotation around a single axis. However, as mentioned, the movement of a TMJ reconstructed by means of a TMJ-TJR prosthesis should predominantly show rotational movement [4]. Since any translational movement cannot be expected to occur in the reconstructed TMJ due to a lack in lateral pterygoid muscle function, we chose to analyse a fixed centre of rotation, even though the Groningen TMJ-TJR allows for some free translation of the neo-disc [8].

When considering a fixed CR of the mandible, placing it more inferiorly should result in increased anterior movement of the associated condyle during mouth opening. Moreover, shifting the CR in a posterior direction should enable relatively more rotation in the coronal plane and, thus, in a more inferior excursion of the condyle [3] (Figure 1).

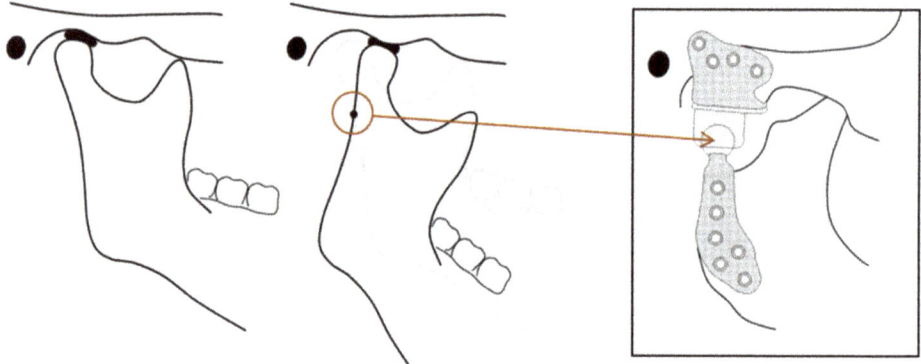

Figure 1. This sketch shows the effect of considering a fixed centre of rotation which is positioned inferior to the centre of the condyle. This lowered centre of rotation mimics the natural translational movement of the condyle whilst merely rotating. The left sketch shows the occlusal mandibular position. Middle shows both the occlusal and maximum opened position of the mandible which is obtained by pure rotation around the dot. The right picture shows the implementation of this effect in the Groningen TMJ-TJR prosthesis, according to the *Groningen Principle*.

Several prior authors have succeeded in analysing the movement of subjects' mandibles by means of tracking them in 2D (sagittal) or 3D [11–18]. Generally, incisal and condylar points are traced during mandibular movement to analyse the mandible's paths of movement, whilst in other cases the mouth opening or closing are described by a path of changing instantaneous centres of rotation throughout the movement. The obtained movement tracking data, or four-dimensional (4D) data, of the mandible could also be used to calculate the CR in a PS manner. This, however, means the patient has to have a physiologically correct movement pattern of the mandible in order to determine these points correctly. Patients who are in need of a TJR of the TMJ often have an affected mouth opening. In such cases, a patient-specific (PS) determined CR of the prosthesis cannot be derived from mandibular movement exercises and so should be determined by alternative means.

The aim of this current study was to develop a 4D-workflow to ascertain the PS mean axis of rotation, or fixed hinge, that mimics the patient's specific physiological mouth opening. The aim was to use this 4D-workflow to find out if the aforementioned prior determined 15 [mm] lowering in CR^3 is still relevant and, if not, to suggest a PS CR location.

2. Materials and Methods

Twenty healthy adult patients who required cone beam computed tomography (CBCT) scanning for 3D virtual surgical planning (VSP) of their bilateral sagittal split osteotomy (BSSO) procedure between January 2020 and December 2021, were asked to volunteer for a 4D-scanning procedure. The inclusion requirements for the 4D-study were the presence of orthodontic brackets and the absence of TMJ dysfunction. Furthermore, the patient should be able to freely move the mandible without pain and other limiting factors. Before commencing with this study's protocol, approval was received from the Medical Ethical Board, file number: METc 2020/355.

The 4D-scanning was performed with a 4D optical tracking module (Planmeca 4D Jaw Motion) installed in a CBCT scanner (Planmeca ProMax, Planmeca, Helsinki, Finland). The resolution of the CBCT images was $0.4 \times 0.4 \times 0.4$ [mm] with a field of view of 230 [mm]. The subjects had to wear a polyamide maxillary frame, which rests on the nasal bridge and ears, and an aluminium mandibular frame rigidly connected to the lower dental arch and orthodontic brackets by means of an easily removable dental bite registration putty (Exabite TT NDS, GC America INC. Alsip, IL, USA). Both the maxillary frame and the mandibular frame accommodated five optical tracer spheres which could be optically recorded by the system (Figure 2). The CBCT scan was performed in maximum dental occlusion with the patient sitting up straight and in natural head position. The field of view was set to include the complete mandible and the maxilla as well as the orbits. Subsequently, movement exercises were carried out and recorded in real time with a frame rate of 24 [Hz].

The recorded experiments comprised five consecutive voluntary maximum mouth opening exercises per patient. The recorded data were exported as transformation matrices describing the transformation from the CBCT image to the mandible position in each frame. The transformation matrices were saved as .xml files and subsequently converted to .xslx format using Excel 2019 (Microsoft, Redmond, Washington, USA) to allow for easier access of the data for further analysis.

The CBCT scan segmentations were performed in the Mimics 22.0 software (Materialise, Leuven, Belgium) and 3D-models of the mandible and maxilla were created. These models were imported into the 3-Matic Medical 15.0 software (Materialise, Leuven, Belgium) to determine the Frankfurt horizontal plane (FHP) and orthogonally positioned midsagittal plane. Parallel to the midsagittal plane, planes were created in the medio-lateral middle of each condyle. These mid-condylar planes were 100×100 [mm] in dimension and triangulated with a maximum edge length of 0.2 [mm]. Subsequently, the mid-condylar planes were merged with the 3D-model of the mandible and exported together with the maxilla model as standard tessellation language (STL) files (Figure 3).

A program was written to develop the JawAnalyser tool in MATLAB R2020a (Mathworks, Natick, Massachusetts, USA) to analyse the recorded 4D-data and to find the instantaneous centre axis of rotation of the moving mandible. The STL models of the maxilla and mandible were imported into this tool together with the subjects' mid-condylar planes and 4D transformation matrix recordings. Start and end frames were chosen manually for each mouth opening, where the start frame was the maximal occlusal position of the mandible prior to the specific mouth opening and the end frame was the maximal open mouth position. The JawAnalyser compares the orientation of the planes of the mandibles' start frame with the opened mandible's planes and finds the point of least translation, and thus maximum rotation, on each plane. These points describe the start and endpoint of the mandible's rotation axis or instantaneous centre of rotation. This 2D technique relies on the Reuleaux method [19] and is translated to 3D by applying two planes to the mandible to find the instantaneous centre of rotation.

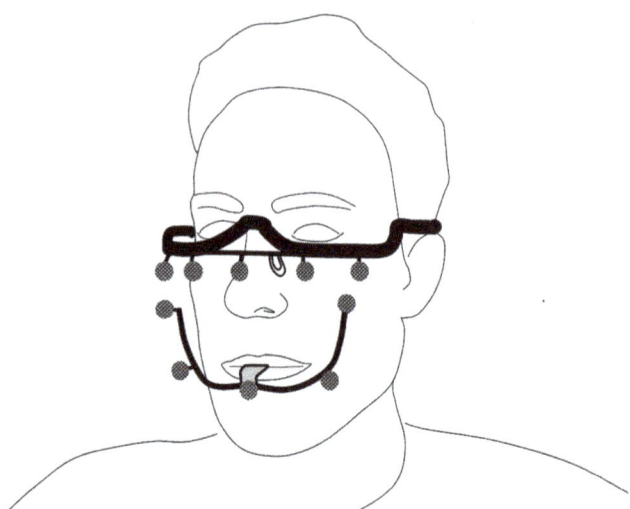

Figure 2. Sketch showing the 4D-CBCT setup. The subject is scanned with CBCT and subsequent 4D optical scanning in one procedure. The subject wears a maxillary frame resting on the nasal bridge and ears and a mandibular frame which is rigidly connected to the dental elements. Both frames are provided with five reflective markers that are visible on both the CBCT imaging and 4D optical tracking.

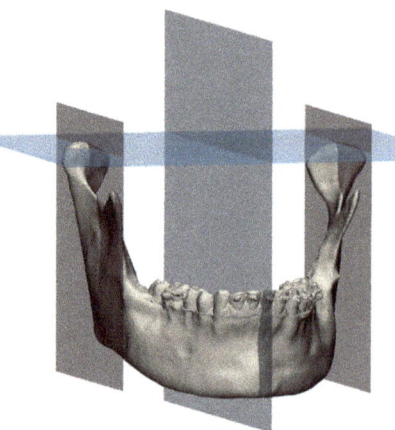

Figure 3. An example of the assigned Frankfurt horizontal plane and matching midsagittal plane (blue). The midsagittal plane was used to create two parallel mid-condylar planes (red), which intersected the condyles in their medio-lateral middle point. These mid-condylar planes were used in the JawAnalyser tool to calculate the patient-specific centres of rotation and, thereby, the patient-specific axis of rotation for the mouth opening.

The accuracy of both the JawAnalyser tool and the entire workflow was validated. The JawAnalyser tool was validated by means of inputting geometries that were manually translated and rotated in space by known quantities and the results of the tool were compared to the known input translation and rotation values.

A phantom model was designed for validation purposes (Figure 4). The entire workflow, starting from the 3D-printing of the phantom, followed by the CBCT imaging, the subsequent 4D-recordings, the segmentations, and the final determined rotation axis, was validated with the aid of this 3D-printed phantom model. This model was based on the dimensions of a human head wearing the maxillary and mandibular tracer set-up, depicted in Figure 2, and was fixed to the CBCT scanner's head-supports. It included the same optical tracer sphere positions as those of our subjects (Figures 2 and 4). The mandible part of the phantom was then rotated 25 degrees around a fixed axis, with ten repetitions, comparable to a mouth opening of approximately 38 [mm]. The rotation axes were then determined using JawAnalyser and compared to the known physical positions of the phantom's rotation axis. The begin and end locations of the rotation axes were determined in the mid-condylar planes and the left and right coordinate sets were registered.

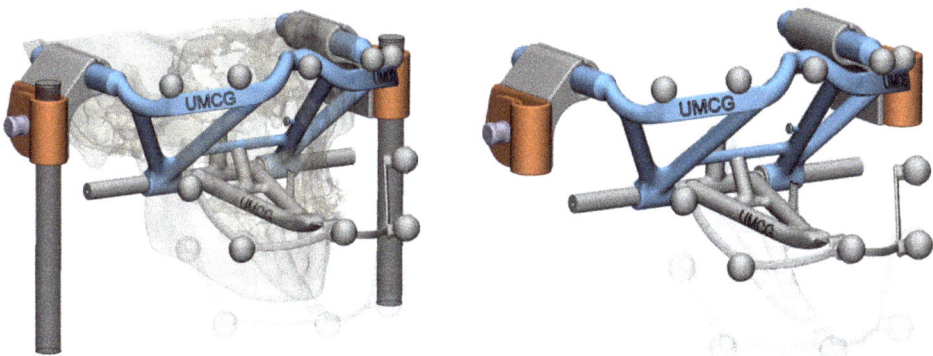

Figure 4. The phantom model that was designed in-house (University Medical Center Groningen /UMCG) for validation of the 4D-workflow. From a subject's scan (**left**), the positions of the optical tracers were determined and the maxillary and mandibular frames were adapted to form a scaffold that could be rigidly connected to the CBCT scanner. The phantom allowed for rotation along the mandibular axis (**right**), resulting in a simulated 25 degrees opened mouth (transparent).

Five pairs of coordinates, indicating the extremities of the axis of rotation for a specific mouth opening, were extracted for each subject from the JawAnalyser tool. The matching start and end frames of these five mouth openings were exported from the JawAnalyser tool as STL files and imported together with the extracted axes of rotation into 3-Matic. Then, all the start frames were matched to the CBCT occlusion mandible position whilst the matching axis of rotation was moved along with its mandible. This was necessary to normalise all the axes positions due to slight changes in occlusal positions. Once brought to the CBCT position, all the rotation axis coordinates were finalised and imported into Excel 2019 to calculate the mean x-, y-, and z-coordinates and one mean axis of rotation per subject.

Using the previously determined mid-condylar planes, a circle was sketched on the cross-section of the condyle. This circle matches the top radius of each condyle and its centre, the centre of condyle (CoC), defines the subject's zero-point, which we used to quantify the position of the patient-specific mean axis of rotation (Figure 5).

The PS CR calculation was carried out for both lateralities in all subjects, resulting in 40 measurements. Regarding each CR, both a Δ x- and Δ y-distance from the CoC were registered in [mm]. The positive x-axis was placed along the FHP in an anterior direction, whilst the positive y-axis was positioned orthogonally to the FHP in a cranial direction. The measured CRs per subject (left and right) were considered independently of each other due to the amount of asymmetry. The data analysis was carried out in in IBM SPSS statistics version 23 (IBM corp., Armonk, NY, USA).

The manual determination of the CoC location was repeated by a second observer for ten condyles (BM and JK). The inter-observer variability calculation was carried out in the SPSS software. The inter-observer variability was supported by calculating the interclass correlation coefficient (ICC), whereby a value of <0.40 is poor, 0.40–0.59 fair, 0.60–0.74 good, and 0.75–1.00 is excellent [20]. This statistical test is an indicator for the reproducibility of our CoC location determination between different observers.

In order to visualise the effect of the calculated mean CR for each patient, points were placed at the inter-incisal point and both CoCs. These points were moved along with the mandible's opening movements so that their coordinates formed paths. These paths, or traces, were then compared to four scenarios. The first was the physiological opening movement we measured with our 4D-tracking system. The second was a simulated opening movement with a pure rotation around the PS calculated mean CR. The third and fourth scenarios were simulations of the left condyle following its physiological path while the right joint was replaced by a fixed CR, either 15 [mm] inferiorly to the CoC or at the calculated PS mean position.

3. Results

Twenty healthy adult subjects were included in this study. These volunteers were 12 males and 8 females, aged from 18 to 53 years, with a mean age of 29. All the subjects had complete natural dentition, wore orthodontic brackets in at least the lower front region, and had no temporomandibular joint dysfunction.

Validation of the JawAnalyser tool resulted in a perfect match between the calculated and input CRs regarding the geometries that were manually rotated and combined, as well as rotated and translated, as is the case in mandibular kinematics. To validate the entire workflow, including the CBCT imaging, the 4D recordings, the segmentations and the final traces, the rotation axes of all ten mouth opening movements were determined for the phantom model. The mean Euclidean error of the start and end coordinates of the rotation axes to the true coordinates of the phantom was 0.81 [mm].

The 40 CR measurements were normally distributed so the mean position was considered to be a relevant indicator. The mean CR of the right-sided joints was located 28.3 [mm] inferiorly and 5.7 [mm] posteriorly, whilst the mean CR of the left joints was located 27.6 [mm] inferiorly and 5.2 [mm] posteriorly to the CoC. When both literalities were combined, the mean CR location was positioned 28 [mm] inferiorly and 5.5 [mm] posteriorly to the CoC. The ranges were ($-45.9/-3.2$ mm) and ($-22.9/+7.5$ mm) for the superoinferior and anteroposterior directions, respectively. The 95% confidence interval of the calculated mean Δ y-distance from the CoC was -22.9 to -33.7 [mm] and -3.1 to -7.8 [mm] for the Δ x-distance. Figure 5 shows a scatter plot of the determined coordinates, indicating the PS positions of the CR, overlaid onto a mandible for reference. Table 1 depicts all the calculated CR positions per subject.

The manual selection of the CoC for both condyles in ten condyles was repeated by a second observer (BM and JK). The inter-observer variation was 1.47 [mm] with an interclass correlation coefficient (two-way mixed) of 0.997, indicating an excellent match for the measurements by both observers.

Patient 19's coordinate tracing throughout the mandibular opening during the four described scenarios is visualised in Figure 6. We chose this patient because of their rather inferior positioned CRs, which pronounces the differences between the four scenarios well.

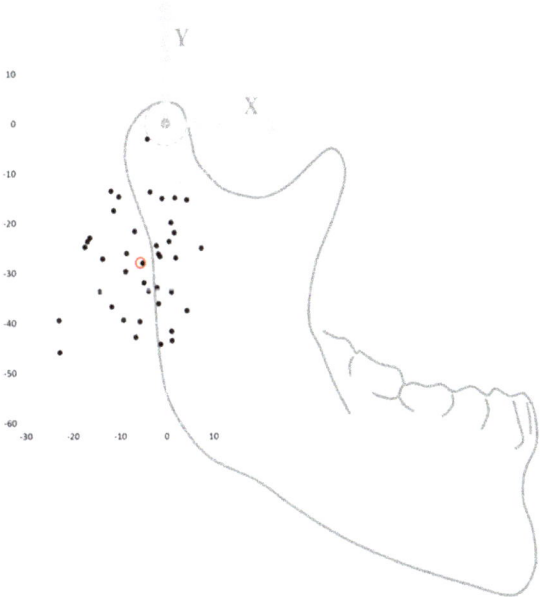

Figure 5. A scatter plot showing the 40 patient-specific centres of rotation coordinates we determined for our cohort (left & right sides). They are overlaid onto a generic mandible for reference, where the (0, 0) point lies in the centre of condyle point (CoC). The red circle indicates the mean measurement, (−5.7, −28.3).

Table 1. All the calculated centre of rotation (CR) positions per subject and per laterality. The delta-Y and delta-X columns show the distance from the patient's specific centre of condyle (CoC) point, which lies in (0, 0). A negative delta-Y value indicates a shift inferiorly of the CoC and a negative delta-X value indicates a shift in the posterior direction.

Patient	Sex	Age	Right CR		Left CR	
			Δ Y	Δ X	Δ Y	Δ X
1	M	19	−39.7	−5.7	−39.4	−9.2
2	M	18	−13.7	−3.4	−14.9	1.9
3	F	53	−13.5	−11.8	−14.7	−10.1
4	F	20	−15.0	−0.8	−25.0	7.5
5	F	19	−33.6	−3.8	−21.7	−6.8
6	F	32	−26.6	−1.3	−28.0	−5.1
7	M	18	−45.9	−22.8	−39.4	−22.9
8	M	25	−3.2	−4.0	−24.5	−2.1
9	F	23	−23.7	−16.7	−24.7	−17.3
10	M	26	−29.7	−8.7	−31.9	−4.8
11	M	18	−23.0	−16.3	−33.7	−14.2
12	F	26	−19.9	1.0	−15.3	4.5
13	F	18	−33.8	1.2	−26.2	−1.6
14	M	46	−41.6	1.2	−43.5	1.2
15	M	47	−27.2	−13.6	−26.0	−8.5
16	F	47	−37.5	4.4	−26.9	2.1
17	M	23	−36.1	−1.7	−32.8	−1.9
18	M	44	−21.9	1.8	−23.7	0.6
19	M	40	−44.2	−1.2	−42.8	−6.7
20	M	29	−36.7	−11.7	−17.5	−11.2
		Mean	−28.3	−5.7	−27.6	−5.2

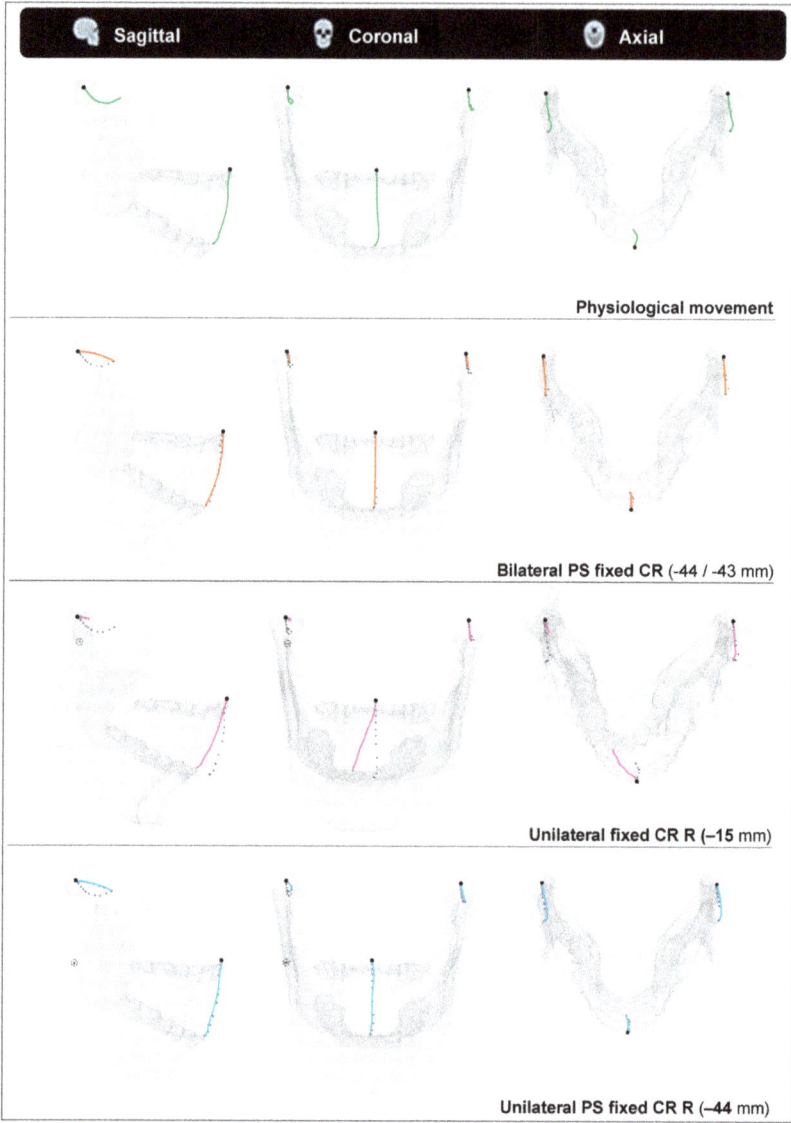

Figure 6. Condylar and incisal point traces describing the mouth opening movement in four different scenarios. Top to bottom: Physiological movement describes the actual recorded movement pattern for this specific subject. Bilateral PS fixed CR describes a simulated mouth opening around the patient-specific (PS) axis of rotation determined with our workflow. Unilateral fixed CR R describes a simulated mouth opening with a fixed centre of rotation (CR) at 15 mm inferior to the centre of condyle (CoC) and the physiological movement of the left condyle. Unilateral PS fixed CR R describes a simulated mouth opening with a fixed CR at the PS determined position, 44 mm inferior to the CoC and the physiological movement of the left condyle. The dotted traces in the three simulated mouth openings indicate the physiological movement traces. Note the severe lateral deviation that occurs when the CR is positioned much closer to the CoC than PS determined.

4. Discussion

The workflow and associated JawAnalyser tool developed in this study serve the purpose of determining the optimal PS fixed axis of rotation. The primary application of such PS rotation axes is in designing PS TMJ-TJRs. None of the commercially available TMJ-TJRs make use of a PS calculated CR in their designs, and their CR positions are based on, e.g., the anatomical condylar position / CoC [21] or on technical limitations, i.e., required minimal thicknesses of the used materials [22]. In the Groningen TMJ-TJR, however, the CR is placed 15 [mm] inferior to the CoC with the aim of mimicking the physiological movement [7]. In this prosthesis, the 15 [mm] CR can be easily substituted by a PS determined value due to its patient-specific design [8,9]. This is naturally within certain boundaries set by the surgical approaches used for implantation.

The PS CRs determined in this study mimic the complex physiological mandibular mouth opening movement, which consists of both translational and rotational movements, by approaching the mouth opening as merely a rotational movement around the PS calculated rotation axis.

By taking all the patients in our cohort into account, we determined the mean position of the CR as being 28 [mm] inferiorly and 5.5 [mm] posteriorly to the CoC. The 95% coincidence intervals for the mean indicate the probability of the majority of the measurements lie within 23 and 34 [mm] inferiorly and 3 to 8 [mm] posteriorly to the CoC. Many prior researchers have studied the kinematics of the mandible [12–18], but the only study which determined a mean CR position that mimicked the physiological mouth opening was the one by van Loon et al. [3]. As mentioned before, they determined an optimal CR of 15 mm inferior to the CoC. Although they did not report specific CRs per subject, they did mention that for the determination of their optimal CR, the physical boundary conditions, i.e., the prosthesis dimensions, were considered as well. This influenced the determination of their optimal centre of location, and therefore, it was not the merely anatomical optimal centre of rotation. Lowering the CR by 15 [mm] with respect to the CoC can already be challenging in some of the smaller patients. Therefore, it does not appear feasible to directly implement the mean of the PS determined CRs to the Groningen TMJ-TJR or in any commercially available prosthesis in most of our entire set of patients. Lindauer et al. also observed a great variation in rotation axes during mouth opening, and they discussed the value of PS determination of CR [23].

After replacing the TMJ with a TJR-prosthesis, it can be assumed that the reconstructed joint will show, postoperatively, rotational movement only [4]. When substituting the physiological movement of the mandible with a mere rotation around the corresponding PS axis of rotation that was calculated with our JawAnalyser, we observed that the inter-incisal point closely matched the physiological trace in all the planes. Although the CoCs matched both the start and end positions, they had an inversely shaped trace when compared to the physiological trace due to the strict rotational movement. When we replaced the right TMJ with a fixed CR located 15 [mm] inferiorly to the CoC, thereby mimicking the replacement of this joint with a Groningen-TMJ-TJR prosthesis, the simulated mouth opening in this particular patient demonstrated an obvious deviation in both the sagittal and coronal planes. The lateral deviation of the inter-incisal point at maximum mouth opening (MMO), however, was more than 12 [mm] in this scenario. The excursion that would have been made by the right condyle if had it not been replaced by the TJR would have been only 6.4 [mm] as opposed to 21.4 [mm] in the measured physiological trace. This indicates that the PS CR for this patient's joint was situated even further inferiorly than 15 [mm]. The latter scenario, where we maintained the left physiological condylar trace and substituted the right joint with a fixed CR at the PS calculated point, showed a perfect match between both the occlusal and MMO positions of the physiological mandible, and the lateral deviation at MMO was non-existent.

The visualised effects of lateral and posterior deviations, as seen in the scenario with unilateral 15 [mm] lowering of a fixed CR (Figure 6), are less pronounced in patients with a smaller mismatch between the applied fixed CR position and the calculated PS CR position.

It should be noted that these deviations are even more pronounced in TJRs with a CR that is positioned higher than 15 [mm], i.e., the Groningen principle. This applies to all commercially available TMJ-TJR prostheses.

This leaves us with three options:

- accept asymmetrical mouth openings and closing movements
- alter the current prosthesis kinematic principles
- adapt the movements of the contralateral joint

Since the latter, entailing operating on and restricting a healthy joint, would be considered unethical, this means only changing the prosthesis concept or accepting a suboptimal mandibular movement. Even though conforming to the PS axis of rotation might not be physically feasible for all cases, knowing the patient's specific axis of rotation is always valuable for predicting the outcome of the TJR procedure and to prepare the patient for the expected outcome.

To illustrate the effect of a mismatched fixed CR on the contralateral healthy joint, we used an exemplary case to compare two condylar position scenarios (Figure 7). The measured physiological MMO position was compared to a simulated MMO in a case of a unilaterally fixed CR (15 [mm] inferior to the CoC), which is comparable with a unilateral TJR. In this particular case, the calculated PS CR is approximately 44 [mm] inferior to the CoC. The contralateral healthy joint completes its full translation, whilst the replaced joint only does approximately a third. As a result of the mismatch between the PS CR and the simulated CR (44 [mm] vs 15 [mm]), the mandible rotates in the axial plane, resulting in a contralateral healthy joint with a condylar seating that is forced to rotate at an 8.2 degree angle. Figure 7 illustrates this rotational error. The patient's measured physiological maximum laterotrusive excursion, throughout the mouth opening, results only in a 1.5-degree angle, which is only 18% of the simulated forced rotation. The effect a forced rotation and change in condylar seating has on the healthy joint, as well as the maximum acceptable forced rotation angles, is still unknown. Additionally, the fact that commercially available prostheses have an even higher CR compared to the 15 [mm] inferiorly placed CR in our case means that, according to the Groningen principle, this effect would have been even greater in those TMJ-TJR prostheses [5,14].

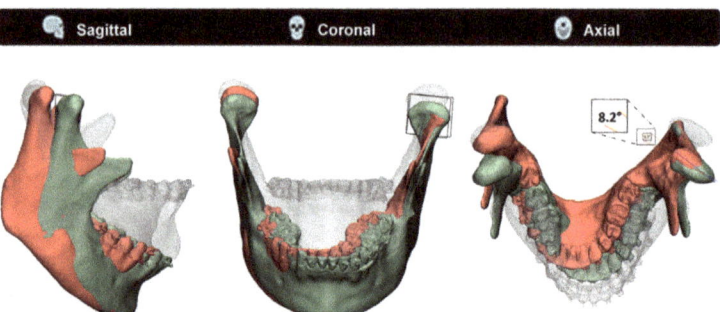

Figure 7. An illustration showing the effect of a wrongly positioned unilateral fixed centre of rotation (CR) simulating a TMJ-TJR prosthesis on the right side, on the healthy contralateral joint. In transparent the occlusal mandibular position is shown. Green indicates the maximum opened mouth according to the recorded physiological data, and red shows the simulated mouth opening according to scenario 'Unilateral fixed CR R (−15 mm)' in Figure 6. The unilateral fixed CR R (−15 mm) scenario is where the left condyle follows the physiological path, whilst the right side has a fixed CR applied too close to the centre of condyle position for this specific patient. Note again the severe lateral deviation of the red mandible and the unnatural rotation this forces on the contralateral healthy joint. In this specific case, the left condyle is forced to rotate an 8.2 degree angle in the axial plane upon opening compared to the physiological opened condyle position.

In patients with restricted mandibular movement, e.g., due to severe unilateral ankylosis, performing a 4D-analysis can be challenging, if not impossible, depending on the severity of the restriction of movement. Furthermore, our proposed workflow would be inapplicable for clinicians who do not have access to 4D techniques. Regarding both situations, it could be worth exploring if the PS CR is related to the morphology of the mandible and fossa and can thus be predicted instead of measured. Among our cohort, we observed that a large portion of the calculated PS CRs lay on or close to the occlusal plane. This observation is supported by prior researchers' findings [24].

In future work, we would like to test the hypothesis that PS CRs can be predicted based on the morphology of the mandible and fossa. Tools that can be applied to test such typical hypotheses are statistical shape modelling (SSM) [25,26] and principal polynomial shape analysis (PPSA) [27]. By using the segmentations of the mandible and fossa together with the calculated PS CRs from our cohort as input for the model, we can make the model predict the PS CRs of mandibles input without 4D data. Further validation of the SSM/PPSA CRs should indicate if there is any relationship between the mandible's morphology and the position of its CRs. However, in order to establish a robust model, we would need to expand our current cohort.

The main limitation of this current study, apart from the relatively small sample size of 20 patients, is the homogeneity of our cohort. Being patients who required CBCT scanning for 3D VSP of their BSSO procedure, all patients in this study had a class II or III occlusion (17 vs. 3). Whether these types of malocclusions have an effect on the movement pattern of the mandible, especially mouth opening, remains unclear, as to the best of our knowledge, this cannot be found in the current literature. Scanning a cohort of control subjects might provide us with these answers, but ethics prevent us from CBCT scanning of healthy subjects.

The strengths, on the other hand, are the fact that our well-validated method turned out a feasible workflow that is not reserved for just BSSO patients. It addresses an issue that seems generally accepted or overlooked and to which more attention should be paid.

5. Conclusions

This study succeeded in developing an accurate 4D-workflow to determine a PS mean axis of rotation that mimics the patient's specific physiological mouth opening. Our results strengthen the conception that PS determination of the CR as, e.g., used in TMJ-TJR prostheses, adds value in regard to mimicking the physiological mouth opening movement. The CRs applied in the commercially available TMJ-TJR prostheses are likely positioned too cranially for the bulk of the population, causing physiologically incorrect mandibular movements. The current PS Groningen TMJ-TJR prosthesis applies a lowered CR of 15 [mm] with respect to the CoC and thereby approaches the physiological movement of the mandible to some extent. The mean optimal CR we determined in this study, 28 [mm] inferior to the CoC, however, implies that 15 [mm] of CR lowering is not sufficient for the bulk of the population. In the Groningen TMJ-TJR and perhaps other commercially available prostheses, the amount of CR can easily be lowered to a PS determined CR within certain boundaries; however, due to technical and surgical constraints this would not be far enough to comply with the PS CRs of the majority of the patients.

Therefore, a change in TMJ-TJR prosthesis concept is necessary for all commercially available prostheses in order to comply with all PS CRs calculated in our study. In the meantime, it seems wise to stick to placing the CR 15 [mm] inferiorly to the CoC, as this already partly mimics the physiological movement, or even beyond, towards 28 [mm], if the patient's anatomy allows this.

Author Contributions: B.B.J.M. conceptualisation, formal analysis, methodology, resources, writing - original draft. M.J.H.W. conceptualisation, software, writing—review and editing. N.B.V.B. conceptualisation, writing—review and editing. J.K.: conceptualisation, methodology, software, supervision, writing—review and editing. F.K.L.S. conceptualisation, investigation, supervision, writing—review and editing. All authors have read and agreed to the published version of the manuscript.

Funding: This research received no external funding.

Institutional Review Board Statement: This study was approved the Medical Ethical Board, file number METc 2020/355.

Informed Consent Statement: Written informed consent was obtained from the patients to publish this paper.

Data Availability Statement: The authors declare that the data supporting the findings of this study are available within the paper.

Acknowledgments: We would like to thank Floris Rotteveel for his efforts in developing the Jaw-Analyser tool and Haye H. Glas and Hylke van der Wel for their support in this. Additionally, we are grateful to the radiologic technician colleagues from our department for their help with the 4D-CBCT recordings.

Conflicts of Interest: The authors declare no conflict of interest.

References

1. Sidebottom, A.J. Current thinking in temporomandibular joint management. *Br. J. Oral Maxillofac. Surg.* **2009**, *47*, 91–94. [CrossRef] [PubMed]
2. Johnson, N.R.; Roberts, M.J.; Doi, S.A.; Batstone, M.D. Total temporomandibular joint replacement prostheses: A systematic review and bias-adjusted meta-analysis. *Int. J. Oral Maxillofac. Surg.* **2017**, *46*, 86–92. [CrossRef] [PubMed]
3. van Loon, J.P.; Falkenstrom, C.H.; de Bont, L.G.; Verkerke, G.J.; Stegenga, B. The theoretical optimal center of rotation for a temporomandibular joint prosthesis: A three-dimensional kinematic study. *J. Dent. Res.* **1999**, *78*, 43–48. [CrossRef]
4. Voiner, J.; Yu, J.; Deitrich, P.; Chafin, C.; Giannakopoulos, H. Analysis of mandibular motion following unilateral and bilateral alloplastic TMJ reconstruction. *Int. J. Oral Maxillofac. Surg.* **2011**, *40*, 569–571. [CrossRef]
5. Wojczynska, A.; Gallo, L.M.; Bredell, M.; Leiggener, C.S. Alterations of mandibular movement patterns after total joint replacement: A case series of long-term outcomes in patients with total alloplastic temporomandibular joint reconstructions. *Int. J. Oral Maxillofac. Surg.* **2019**, *48*, 225–232. [CrossRef]
6. van Loon, J.P.; Otten, E.; Falkenstrom, C.H.; de Bont, L.G.; Verkerke, G.J. Loading of a unilateral temporomandibular joint prosthesis: A three-dimensional mathematical study. *J. Dent. Res.* **1998**, *77*, 1939–1947. [CrossRef]
7. van Loon, J.P.; de Bont, L.G.; Stegenga, B.; Spijkervet, F.K.; Verkerke, G.J. Groningen temporomandibular joint prosthesis. Development and first clinical application. *Int. J. Oral Maxillofac. Surg.* **2002**, *31*, 44–52. [CrossRef]
8. Merema, B.J.; Kraeima, J.; Witjes, M.J.H.; van Bakelen, N.B.; Spijkervet, F.K.L. Accuracy of fit analysis of the patient-specific Groningen temporomandibular joint prosthesis. *Int. J. Oral Maxillofac. Surg.* **2021**, *50*, 538–545. [CrossRef]
9. Kraeima, J.; Merema, B.J.; Witjes, M.J.H.; Spijkervet, F.K.L. Development of a patient-specific temporomandibular joint prosthesis according to the Groningen principle through a cadaver test series. *J. Craniomaxillofac. Surg.* **2018**, *46*, 779–784. [CrossRef]
10. Falkenström, C.H. Biomechanical Design of a Total Temporomandibular Joint Replacement. Ph.D. Thesis, University of Twente, Enschede, The Netherlands, 1993.
11. Hall, R.E. An analysis of the work and ideas of investigators and authors of relations and movements of the mandible. *J. Am. Dent. Assoc.* **1929**, *16*, 1642–1693. [CrossRef]
12. Ahn, S.J.; Tsou, L.; Antonio Sanchez, C.; Fels, S.; Kwon, H.B. Analyzing center of rotation during opening and closing movements of the mandible using computer simulations. *J. Biomech.* **2015**, *48*, 666–671. [CrossRef] [PubMed]
13. Gallo, L.M.; Airoldi, G.B.; Airoldi, R.L.; Palla, S. Description of Mandibular Finite Helical Axis Pathways in Asymptomatic Subjects. *J. Dent. Res.* **1997**, *76*, 704–713. [CrossRef]
14. Wojczyńska, A.; Leiggener, C.; Bredell, M.; Ettlin, D.; Erni, S.; Gallo, L.; Colombo, V. Alloplastic total temporomandibular joint replacements: Do they perform like natural joints? Prospective cohort study with a historical control. *Int. J. Oral Maxillofac. Surg.* **2016**, *45*, 1213–1221.
15. Chen, X. The instantaneous center of rotation during human jaw opening and its significance in interpreting the functional meaning of condylar translation. *Am. J. Phys. Anthropol.* **1998**, *106*, 35–46. [CrossRef]
16. Leader, J.K.; Boston, J.R.; Debski, R.E.; Rudy, T.E. Mandibular kinematics represented by a non-orthogonal floating axis joint coordinate system. *J. Biomech.* **2003**, *36*, 275–281. [CrossRef]
17. Leiggener, C.S.; Erni, S.; Gallo, L.M. Novel approach to the study of jaw kinematics in an alloplastic TMJ reconstruction. *Int. J. Oral Maxillofac. Surg.* **2012**, *41*, 1041–1045. [CrossRef]
18. Chen, C.-C.; Lin, C.-C.; Hsieh, H.-P.; Fu, Y.-C.; Chen, Y.-J.; Lu, T.-W. In vivo three-dimensional mandibular kinematics and functional point trajectories during temporomandibular activities using 3d fluoroscopy. *Dentomaxillofac. Radiol.* **2021**, *50*, 20190464. [CrossRef]
19. Moorehead, J.D.; Montgomery, S.C.; Harvey, D.M. Instant center of rotation estimation using the Reuleaux technique and a Lateral Extrapolation technique. *J. Biomech.* **2003**, *36*, 1301–1307. [CrossRef]

20. Cicchetti, D. Guidelines, Criteria, and Rules of Thumb for Evaluating Normed and Standardized Assessment Instrument in Psychology. *Psychol. Assess.* **1994**, *6*, 284–290. [CrossRef]
21. Zheng, J.; Chen, X.; Jiang, W.; Zhang, S.; Chen, M.; Yang, C. An innovative total temporomandibular joint prosthesis with customized design and 3D printing additive fabrication: A prospective clinical study. *J. Transl. Med.* **2019**, *17*, 4. [CrossRef]
22. Quinn, P.D. Lorenz Prosthesis. In *Oral and Maxillofacial Surgery Clinics of North America*; Elsevier: Amsterdam, The Netherlands, 2000; Volume 12, pp. 93–104.
23. Lindauer, S.J.; Sabol, G.; Isaacson, R.J.; Davidovitch, M. Condylar movement and mandibular rotation during jaw opening. *Am. J. Orthod. Dentofac. Orthop.* **1995**, *107*, 573–577. [CrossRef]
24. Terhune, C.E.; Iriarte-Diaz, J.; Taylor, A.B.; Ross, C.F. The instantaneous center of rotation of the mandible in nonhuman primates. *Integr. Comp. Biol.* **2011**, *51*, 320–332. [CrossRef] [PubMed]
25. Yang, Y.M.; Rueckert, D.; Bull, A.M. Predicting the shapes of bones at a joint: Application to the shoulder. *Comput. Methods Biomech. Biomed. Engin.* **2008**, *11*, 19–30. [CrossRef] [PubMed]
26. Vlachopoulos, L.; Lüthi, M.; Carrillo, F.; Gerber, C.; Székely, G.; Fürnstahl, P. Restoration of the Patient-Specific Anatomy of the Proximal and Distal Parts of the Humerus: Statistical Shape Modeling Versus Contralateral Registration Method. *J. Bone Jt. Surg. Am.* **2018**, *100*, e50. [CrossRef]
27. Duquesne, K.; Nauwelaers, N.; Claes, P.; Audenaert, E. Principal polynomial shape analysis: A non-linear tool for statistical shape modeling. *Comput. Methods Programs Biomed.* **2022**, *220*, 106812. [CrossRef]

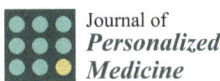

Review

Personalized Medicine Workflow in Post-Traumatic Orbital Reconstruction

Juliana F. Sabelis [1,*], Ruud Schreurs [1,2], Harald Essig [3], Alfred G. Becking [1] and Leander Dubois [1]

1. Department of Oral and Maxillofacial Surgery, Amsterdam University Medical Centre (UMC), AMC, Academic Center for Dentistry Amsterdam (ACTA), Meibergdreef 9, 1105 AZ Amsterdam, The Netherlands
2. Department of Oral and Maxillofacial Surgery, Radboud University Medical Centre Nijmegen, Geert Grooteplein Zuid 10, 6525 GA Nijmegen, The Netherlands
3. Department Oral & Maxillofacial Surgery, University Hospital, Frauenklinikstrasse 24, 8091 Zurich, Switzerland
* Correspondence: j.f.sabelis@amsterdamumc.nl

Abstract: Restoration of the orbit is the first and most predictable step in the surgical treatment of orbital fractures. Orbital reconstruction is keyhole surgery performed in a confined space. A technology-supported workflow called computer-assisted surgery (CAS) has become the standard for complex orbital traumatology in many hospitals. CAS technology has catalyzed the incorporation of personalized medicine in orbital reconstruction. The complete workflow consists of diagnostics, planning, surgery and evaluation. Advanced diagnostics and virtual surgical planning are techniques utilized in the preoperative phase to optimally prepare for surgery and adapt the treatment to the patient. Further personalization of the treatment is possible if reconstruction is performed with a patient-specific implant and several design options are available to tailor the implant to individual needs. Intraoperatively, visual appraisal is used to assess the obtained implant position. Surgical navigation, intraoperative imaging, and specific PSI design options are able to enhance feedback in the CAS workflow. Evaluation of the surgical result can be performed both qualitatively and quantitatively. Throughout the entire workflow, the concepts of CAS and personalized medicine are intertwined. A combination of the techniques may be applied in order to achieve the most optimal clinical outcome. The goal of this article is to provide a complete overview of the workflow for post-traumatic orbital reconstruction, with an in-depth description of the available personalization and CAS options.

Keywords: patient-specific implants; orbital reconstruction; computer-assisted surgery; surgical navigation; additive manufacturing

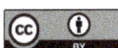

1. Introduction

The orbit is an inward-projecting bony structure in the shape of a cone (or pyramid) at the transition between midface and skull base [1–3]. The base of the orbit, the orbital rim, is composed of thick bone; in contrast, the orbit's inner walls are thin bony structures. The orbit provides the casing for the soft-tissue structures associated with the visual (motor) system: neurovascular structures, connective tissue, ocular muscles, and the globe [4,5].

With its central position and thin bony walls, the orbit is probably the most vulnerable part of the facial skeleton [1,2]. Two possible theories of orbital fracture pathogenesis have been suggested. The buckling theory suggests that the energy of a traumatic impact on the orbital rim after blunt-force trauma is propagated to the thin inner walls and leads to a fracture in these weaker structures [6–8]. Hydraulic theory considers increased pressure after impact on the globe and orbital contents as the main reason for orbital wall fractures. The exact nature and specifics of a fracture may be explained by a combination of both mechanisms [7].

The orbital volume may be increased, and soft tissue may be displaced into the adjacent sinuses due to the impact or the dislocation of supporting bony structures. The globe's position may be displaced after trauma, for instance, with inward displacement (enophthalmos) or inferior displacement (hypoglobus). The orbital soft tissue may be affected by the traumatic impact as well. The structural integrity and functional capacities of connective tissue or extraocular muscles may be disrupted, resulting in a disturbance of ocular motility and double vision (diplopia). The location and type of the impact, in combination with the amount of energy transferred to the orbit's bony structures and orbital soft tissue, are responsible for the heterogeneity in clinical presentation.

There is an ongoing debate on the indication of surgical reconstruction, and systematic reviews have not been able to provide evidence-supported guidelines [9–11]. Some advocate a radical approach to prevent clinical symptoms [12], while others choose a more conservative approach with a delayed surgery if clinical symptoms develop [13]. Indication for reconstruction remains a subjective decision in most cases, depending on the surgeon and patient characteristics. The surgical management of orbital fractures focuses on the repositioning the orbital contents and the globe and reinstating the structural support to recover ocular function. Restoration of the orbit is the first and most predictable step in the surgical treatment of orbital fractures [14,15].

Nowadays, titanium mesh implants have become the preferred biomaterial for the surgical reconstruction of the orbit. Titanium implants can be categorized into flat implants, preformed implants, and patient-specific implants (PSIs). Flat implants are manually shaped and trimmed by the surgeon. A generic or individual model of the (mirrored) orbit may aid in the molding process. Preformed implants have a predefined shape, based on a model of the average orbit [10,16]. Patient-specific implants (PSIs) are designed on an individual basis for the patient and are subsequently produced through additive manufacturing.

The soft tissue's intricate architecture and the proximity to vital structures pose surgical challenges in orbital reconstruction [17,18]. Orbital reconstruction is keyhole surgery performed in a confined space. This contributes to limited visualization, which is further enhanced by protruding fat. The margin of error is small: an incorrectly positioned implant may have significant implications for the clinical outcome and the patient's quality of life, and it is considered a ground for revision surgery in the literature [19,20]. Medical technology has been incorporated in the clinical workflow of orbital reconstructions to reduce the risk of implant malpositioning [21].

This technology-supported workflow, called computer-assisted surgery (CAS), has become the standard for complex orbital traumatology in many hospitals [22]. The introduction of CAS has also enabled personalization of the treatment: treatment planning is customized to fit the options and needs of the patient, and intraoperative guidance is adjusted to the anatomical possibilities. The main aim of this article is to provide a complete overview of the (CAS) workflow for orbital reconstruction, with an in-depth description of the techniques embedded in the workflow and with a special focus on treatment personalization through patient-specific implant design.

2. Post-Traumatic Orbital Reconstruction Workflow

The conventional workflow of post-traumatic orbital reconstruction and possible CAS techniques are illustrated in Figure 1. The individual phases are explained in detail in the following paragraphs.

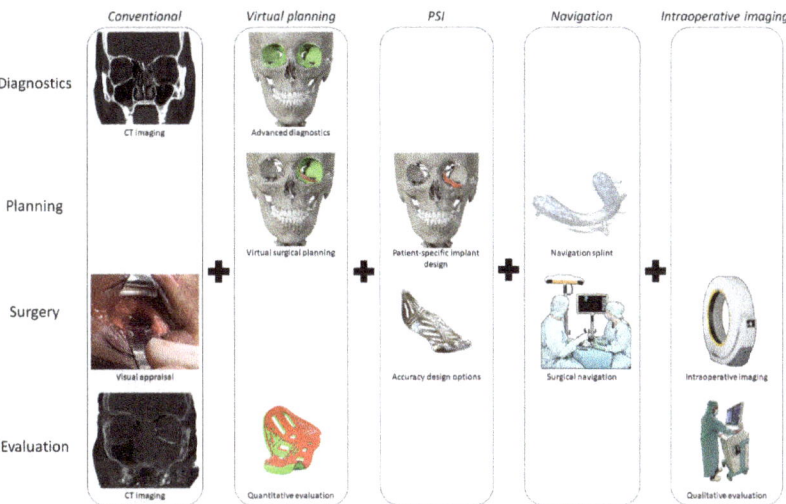

Figure 1. Schematic overview of the technological possibilities within the orbital reconstruction workflow. Chronologically, a clinical workflow consists of diagnostics, planning, surgery, and evaluation. In the conventional workflow, the surgeon is dependent on clinical assessment and preoperative imaging, visual appraisal during surgery and postoperative imaging for evaluation. CAS consists of several techniques that may be combined and affect one or multiple workflow stages. Several CAS technologies may be combined.

2.1. Diagnostics

A thorough clinical and radiographic evaluation of the patient is essential to determine the optimal treatment. Clinical evaluation should at least assess the amount of globe displacement and the degree of double vision. The Hertel exophthalmometer is the simplest tool to quantitatively measure the relative ventrodorsal globe position [23]. It is the current gold standard despite the known limitations, such as the asymmetry of lateral orbital rims, the compression of soft tissue, and the lack of a uniform technique [23,24]. There are no readily available reproducible tools for measuring the relative craniocaudal globe position [25]. It is assessed by the Hirschberg test, which evaluates the light reflex centered on each pupil to reveal vertical asymmetry [26]. Alternative methods have been proposed to quantify globe position differences based on imaging, but these have not been broadly implemented [23,27].

One of the difficulties in clinical decision-making is to address the most common complaint in orbital fractures: diplopia. It is challenging to find the actual cause of diplopia; in most cases, it is caused by a restriction of ocular motility. Ocular motility can be disturbed by impingement or the entrapment of the ocular muscles and surrounding soft tissue, but also by muscle edema, muscle injury, hemorrhage, emphysema, or motor nerve palsy. In a trauma setting, orthoptic measurements may be challenging to perform due to logistics, limited mobility of the patient, or considerable periorbital swelling. Absolute restrictions, as seen in trapdoor fractures, need to be treated shortly after the trauma. Ocular motility deficits with different etiology may improve or resolve over time, and surgery might not be indicated. In these cases, it is advisable to perform several orthoptic assessments over time to monitor spontaneous improvement. Moreover, the orthoptist may be able to differentiate between possible causes of double vision through repeated measurements [9,28].

Computed tomography (CT) is the modality of choice for radiographic evaluation because of the superior visualization of bony structures. The size and extent of the fracture may be estimated or measured in the coronal, sagittal, or axial plane. Considering that the bone is paper-thin in certain areas, a maximum slice thickness of 1.0 mm is essential for evaluation. In individual cases, the evaluation of soft-tissue changes may become important. Shape alterations of the inferior rectus muscle have been reported to affect delayed or postoperative enophthalmos [29–31] and may affect treatment decisions [10]. In addition, herniation of the orbital soft tissue might be an indication for surgical reconstruction. Magnetic resonance imaging (MRI) provides superior soft-tissue contrast compared to CT and is more sensitive for identifying extraocular muscle or periorbital fat entrapment [32,33]. Nevertheless, the acquisition of an MRI is not part of the standard imaging protocol for orbital trauma [13]. This may change in the future, considering that all subsequent treatment steps benefit from optimizing the information collection in the diagnostics phase.

2.2. Advanced Diagnostics

Advanced diagnostics aim to maximize the information extracted from the available image data. For this purpose, the CT scan is imported into the virtual surgical planning software. The CT scan is subdivided into voxels (3D pixels), each with a grayscale value corresponding to the X-ray absorption within that volume. These voxels may be segmented (grouped) based on the tissue type or anatomical structure they belong to. Anatomical structures of interest in orbital trauma are the orbit, orbital cavity, and possibly surrounding bony structures such as the zygomatic complex. The segmentation is visualized as an overlay in the multi-planar view and as a 3D model. Additional information may be collected through quantification (e.g., volume measurement), or manipulation (e.g., mirroring) of the segmented anatomy (illustrated in Figure 2). The unaffected contralateral orbit and orbital cavity can provide a reference for the affected orbit in unilateral fractures, which provides insight into the extent of the fracture and displacement of orbital walls or surrounding bony structures. The volume of the affected orbit can be compared to the unaffected healthy side to determine the relative volume change, since it has been proven that the orbits are highly symmetrical [33]. These volumetric changes can be incorporated into the treatment plan [34]. Information may also be extracted from multiple image sets. Image fusion allows aligning multiple datasets of the same modality over time or image sets from different modalities. The image sets can be simultaneously visualized and evaluated after image fusion. The segmentation process can also be based on information from multiple fused modalities.

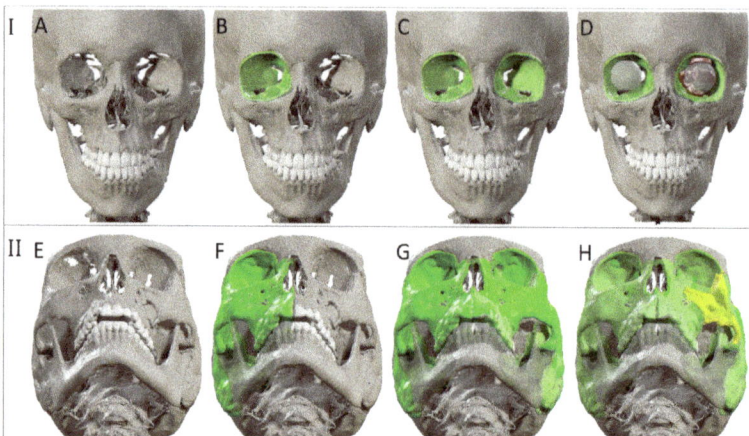

Figure 2. Advanced diagnostics for two cases. I: Solitary orbital reconstruction (**A**–**D**). (**A**) Visualization of the 3D bone surface model. (**B**) Segmentation of the unaffected orbit. (**C**) Mirroring of the segmented orbit to the affected, contralateral side. (**D**) Visualization of additional structures, such as the globe and eye muscles. II: Zygomatic complex fracture (**E**–**H**). (**E**) Visualization of the 3D bone surface model. (**F**) Segmentation of the unaffected side. (**G**) Mirroring of the segmentation to the affected, contralateral side. (**H**) Visualization of the zygomatic complex displacement.

2.3. Virtual Surgical Planning

Virtual surgical planning (VSP) is a simulation of the actual surgery on the imaging data [35]. It is based on information gathered in the previous treatment stages. The exact content of the virtual surgical planning depends on the type of implant. If a flat mesh plate is used, the virtual models of the mirrored orbit and affected orbit can be exported and 3D printed to serve as individual bending template(s) for molding the flat mesh.

In the preformed implant setting, the stereolithographic model (STL) of a preformed implant is imported into the planning environment to perform a virtual reconstruction of the affected orbit. The implant's fitting potential is evaluated and its optimal position for an accurate reconstruction of the pretraumatized anatomy is simulated. The potential of VSP in the preformed implant setting is thus highly dependent on the willingness of the implant manufacturers to provide STLs of their preformed implants. In modern planning software, the implant may be automatically aligned to another virtual model, for instance, the mirrored orbit. Manual adjustments could be necessary to prevent interferences with the bone and ensure the orbital defect is covered, with adequate implant support on the dorsal ledge and fixation possibility on the infraorbital rim.

The implant may be virtually trimmed to simulate the cutting of medial or posterior parts of the implant. The surgery can be simulated multiple times in the virtual surgical planning, with different implant types and sizes (Figure 3). This enables comparison between preformed implant options and substantiated decision making before surgery. The number of try-ins in virtual planning is limitless without consequences for the patient, in contrast to try-ins during actual surgery. Establishing the optimal position in virtual planning provides the surgeon with intraoperative feedback, which could reduce the operating time and extent of manipulation inside the orbit during surgery [36].

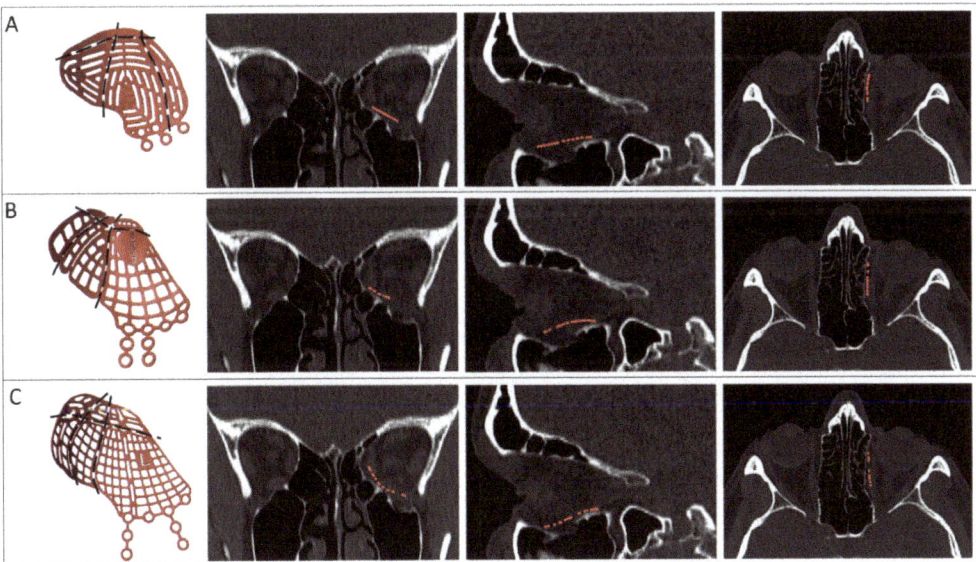

Figure 3. Virtual fitting of different preformed implants in a solitary orbital fracture. Three-dimensional models of the preformed implants of KLS Martin (**A**), Synthes (**B**) and Stryker (**C**) are visualized with potential cutting lines (black lines) in the first column. The implants are virtually positioned (red contour) and the fit is evaluated in the coronal, sagittal, and axial slices. Important considerations are adequate support (on the posterior ledge, on the medial wall and on the infraorbital rim) and a lack of interference with bone.

2.4. Patient-Specific Implant Design

Reconstructing the orbit with a PSI is the ultimate step of individualization for orbital reconstruction. A PSI is virtually modelled from scratch, using information from the (advanced) diagnostics phase and exported virtual models. In dedicated design software, a prototype implant is generated. The prototype is imported into the virtual surgical planning and its fit is evaluated. The position of the prototype is not adjusted in the virtual surgical planning to improve the fit, but the design of the prototype is adjusted and the novel prototype is reimported. Even though the design of a PSI is not set in stone by protocols, various design considerations have been described in the literature. An overview of options is summarized in Table 1. This overview is not comprehensive, and novel design options are regularly introduced in the literature.

Table 1. List of different design considerations as reported in the literature.

Design Consideration	Effect on	Options	References	Notes
Thickness	Positioning, stability	0.3 mm	[22,37,38]	
Atraumatic cord	Positioning, stability	Present	[37,39,40]	
		Absent	[38,41,42]	
Grid	Clinical symptoms	Horizontal Squares Porous	[22,37,40,43] [38,39,41,44] [42,45,46]	
Support	Stability, accuracy	Three points	[22]	Infraorbital rim, medial wall, posterior ledge
			[38]	Anteromedial, anterolateral, posterior
		Ledge	[37,40,43]	Inverted shovel design
		Lateral posterior wall	[43]	Stabilizer for self-centering implant
Extension	Accuracy	Orbital rim	[22,42,44,46–48]	
		Lateral posterior wall	[43]	
		Specific bone features	[45]	
Anterior elevation	Clinical symptoms		[22]	Rim elevation to correct hypoglobus
Overcorrection	Clinical symptoms	Location	[22]	Posterior to bulbus
			[49]	Orbital floor elevated in sagittal relation
		Amount	[22]	Based on clinical findings, advanced diagnostics
			[38]	Slight overcorrection
			[50]	Same amount in cubic cm as mm enophthalmos
		Intraoperatively	[51]	Spacers
Navigation	Accuracy	Markers	[22,37–39,52]	Eminence lacrimal foramen [38]
		Vectors	[37,40,43]	
Fixation	Stability	Absent	[38,44,48]	
		Present	[22,37,39,40,42, 46,47,53]	Eccentric screw alters implant position [47] Fix implant if form stable [40]
Fixation re-use	Accuracy	Re-used screw hole	[54]	Only in secondary reconstruction
Multi-piece	Positioning, stability, accuracy	Lazy-S	[42,47,49]	
		Interlocking	[46,48,55,56]	

Design considerations can be categorized based on their intended effect: stability, positioning ease, accuracy of implant positioning or alleviation of clinical symptoms. The size and shape of the implant are dependent on the extent of the defect. The defect should be covered by the implant and its shape should reflect the intended reconstruction of the affected orbital walls. Support on existing bony structures is taken into account to ensure the stability of the reconstruction. Analogous to the preformed implants, support is most often found at three points in the orbit [22,38]. Fixation is recommended to ensure a stable position of the PSI [39,40]. Possible screw positions can be assessed in virtual planning, factoring in the patient's anatomy and local bone quality. The thickness of the implant and implementation of an atraumatic cord around the edge are considerations that affect both the stability of the implant and the positioning ease during surgery. Due to additive-manufactured titanium's rigidity, an implant thickness of 0.3 mm in combination with an atraumatic cord results in a good balance between rigidity and positioning ease.

The accuracy of implant positioning can be controlled by extensions over unaffected bony pillars. A compelling fit is created by the extension(s) of the implant over bony structures. An infraorbital rim extension limits rotation and translation in the anteroposterior direction [47]. Additional flanges to the posterior lateral wall may be implemented to prevent unwanted implant movement [43]. Screw positions from fixation material from a previous reconstruction can be re-used in secondary reconstruction to provide guidance and thus improve the accuracy of the implant positioning [54]. Another design option is to incorporate navigation markers and vectors, which can enhance the interpretation of feedback from the intraoperative navigation system.

The last category, clinical symptoms, deals with the correction of globe displacement. The orbital volume is corrected to alleviate globe displacement, but the volume may be overcorrected to counteract fat atrophy and the anticipated iatrogenic loss of soft tissue [57]. The amount of overcorrection might be subjectively determined during surgery, by inserting additional spacers [51], or it may be fully integrated into the design of the PSI, posterior to the equator of the bulbus [22,38,50]. On the other hand, hypoglobus is the result of caudal displacement of the infra-orbital rim. An anterior elevation corresponding to the amount of downward displacement of the orbital rim may alleviate hypoglobus (Figure 4). The grid of the PSI can be designed with different techniques: using a large horizontal pattern to maximize drainage [37,40,43], or a more porous arrangement [42,45,46]. The multitude of design options and manual design leads to a wide range of possible PSI shapes (Figure 5).

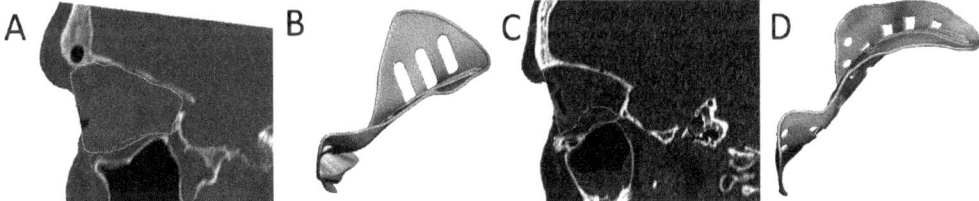

Figure 4. Examples of two patient-specific implant designs with overcorrection (red contour) of the mirrored orbital volume (yellow contour). The first patient-specific implant is designed with an anterior elevation at the infra-orbital rim to compensate for the asymmetry in globe position (**A**,**B**). The second patient-specific implant is designed with a large overcorrection for an anophthalmic socket reconstruction (**C**,**D**).

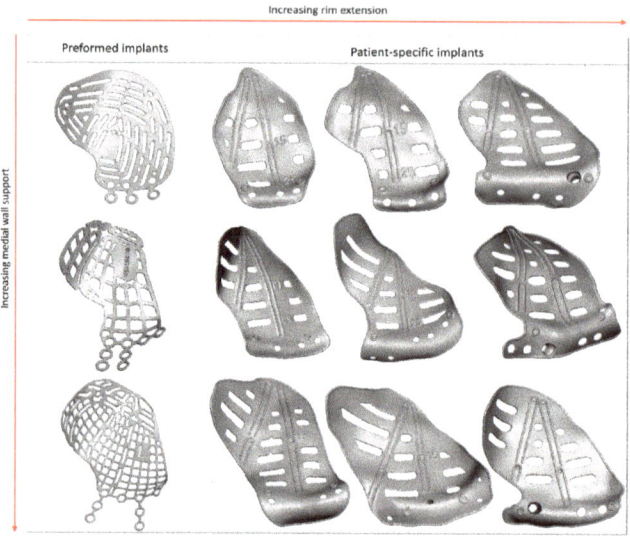

Figure 5. Different shapes of the available preformed implants and patient-specific implants are illustrated. There is a wide variety in shapes in the patient-specific implants. From left to right the rim extension is increased. From top to bottom the medial wall support is increased.

The PSI design can be adapted to facilitate the reconstruction of multi-wall defects, for example, through the application of multiple PSIs (Figure 6). This enables a reconstruction that covers the entire defect while limiting the size of the PSI and, in turn, the required incision [46,55]. Depending on the connection used, it also provides the opportunity to create artificial support and relative feedback. A PSI that solely reconstructs the orbit will not suffice in cases with concomitant fractures of the surrounding bony structures. Repositioning the surrounding bone may be required in addition to the orbital reconstruction. Additional design options are available to gain feedback from PSIs on the subsequent reconstruction steps in these more extensive cases. An example of this is embedding the desired position of the zygomatic complex in the PSI design to facilitate correct repositioning [54].

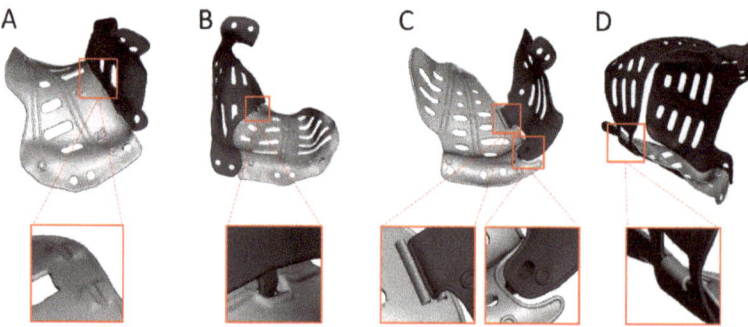

Figure 6. Patient-specific implant design for multi-wall cases. (**A**) Ridges on the orbital floor implant provide relative feedback for the positioning of the lateral wall implant. (**B**) Patrix–matrix connection to connect a medial wall and orbital floor implant. (**C**) The orbital floor implant with medial wall extension is connected to a lateral wall implant dorsally with ridges and anteriorly with a puzzle connection. (**D**) Four-wall reconstruction with a hook-and-bar connection for additional support for the orbital floor implant.

2.5. Intraoperative Feedback

During surgery, the surgeon aims to position the implant as closely as possible to the ideal position that was established in the VSP. The availability of the VSP provides intraoperative feedback that improves the result of the reconstruction [35]. Additional types of feedback are available to aid in the accurate positioning of the implant (summarized in Table 2). The design options relating to implant positioning ensure static feedback through the unique and compelling fit of the PSI (Figure 7). In secondary cases, the re-use of screw positions from the primary reconstruction will also help to find the planned position.

Table 2. Different feedback methods available in the operation room.

Feedback Method	Static/Dynamic
Virtual surgical planning	Static
Compelling fit patient-specific implant	Static
Fixation re-use	Static
Navigation	Dynamic
Markers and vectors	Dynamic
Intraoperative imaging	Static

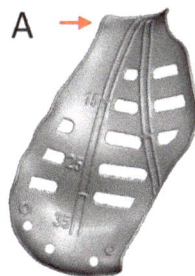
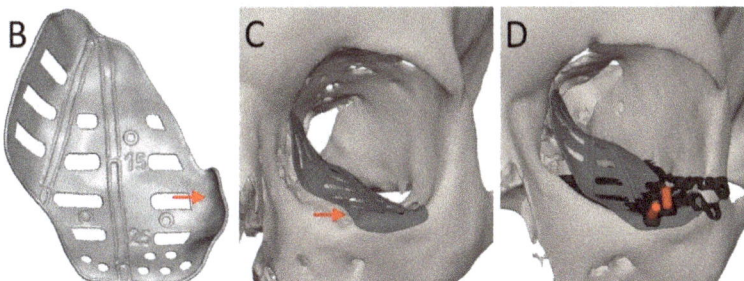

Figure 7. Illustration of the different feedback methods.). Markers and vectors are visualized in (**A**) and (**B**). Compelling fit of the patient-specific implant design is indicated with red arrows (**A–C**) Segmentation of screw holes of the previous reconstruction are illustrated in red (**D**) and the previous implant in dark grey.

Surgical navigation may be utilized to provide dynamic feedback on the implant position. During the registration for surgical navigation, the patient's position in the operating room (OR) is linked to the preoperative imaging data in the virtual surgical planning. Several registration methods are available: soft-tissue registration, bone-anchored fiducials, and surgical splints [56,58]. Splint registration methods used to require repeated radiographic imaging with the fiducial splint in place, but the fusion of intraoral scan data in the advanced diagnostics phase allows the fabrication of a registration splint without additional radiologic imaging [59]. The splint is designed on the individual patient's dentition and carries fiducials that can be indicated virtually in the planning software and physically in the OR.

After registration, the navigation pointer's position in the patient is visualized in the virtual surgical planning on the navigation system's screen. This provides the surgeon with feedback on the position of the pointer, representing the position of the indicated location (a specific spot on the implant's surface). The quality and interpretability of the feedback may be enhanced through navigation markers embedded in the design [39,52]. The markers are indicated in the VSP as navigation landmarks and used as a reference in the OR. If the surgeon positions the pointer in the navigation marker on the implant, visual and quantitative feedback about the pointer's position compared to the landmark is provided.

2.6. Evaluation

Intraoperative imaging of the patient after implant positioning is highly recommended, since the realized implant position can be qualitatively evaluated. If the surgeon is not satisfied with the position, the implant can be repositioned in the same surgical setting, preventing a revision surgery. For a complete quantitative evaluation of the surgical result, the scan can be reconstructed and fused with the VSP. The planned position of the implant can be compared to the achieved position of the implant to enable an objective assessment (Figure 8). Differences between planned and realized position can be quantified in three dimensions and expressed as rotations (roll, pitch and yaw) and translations (x, y and z) [60]. Additionally, the volumetric difference between the reconstructed and unaffected or planned orbit may be assessed. Post-operative CT-scans are indicated if intra-operative CT is not acquired (or offered incomplete information), or if clinical considerations in the follow-up period necessitate additional imaging.

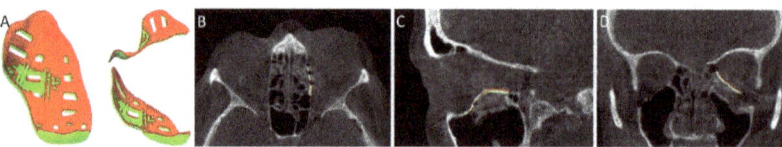

Figure 8. Illustration of an evaluation. (**A**) Three-dimensional model of the planned patient-specific implant (red) and the realized patient-specific implant (green) viewed from different perspectives. (**B–D**) Axial, sagittal, and coronal view of the postoperative computed tomography scan with the planned contour of the patient-specific implant in red.

An optimally positioned orbital implant is no guarantee for a perfect clinical outcome. Restoration of the globe position can be relatively well achieved with a PSI, even in secondary reconstructions [22]. It is more complex to treat diplopia, as it involves the mechanical mobility of the eye, combined visual perception, and processing in the visual cortex. Visual processing may (partially) adapt over time. At discharge, the patient is informed that double vision will be experienced for the first 10–14 days, possibly longer. Ocular motility can be improved by training the extraocular muscles to prevent scarring and anticipate fibrosis [61]. Instructions are provided to mobilize the eye as much as possible: monocular orthoptic exercises six times per day for 6–12 weeks to prevent adhesions and stimulate a reduction in orbital soft tissue swelling, especially for the extraocular muscles. This protocol positively affects clinical improvement in both primary and secondary cases [13,22,47].

3. Discussion

Surgical complexity and the fact that an inappropriate reconstruction potentially leads to an adverse outcome have led to the parallel incorporation of computer-assisted surgery and personalized medicine in the orbital reconstruction workflow. Although both concepts aim to optimize treatment outcome, their rationale differs. CAS centralizes medical technology to improve the predictability and accuracy of all treatment stages, but various steps have been standardized and can be considered independent of the patient. CAS has catalyzed the incorporation of personalized medicine in orbital reconstruction: virtual surgical planning technology enables surgical preparation, implant selection, and the simulation of the desired implant position based on the individual's characteristics. The concepts are considerably intertwined in PSI reconstruction, and mutual interactions can be discerned. Personalization of the implant design is directly affected by information gathered in the preoperative CAS stage, and tailoring the implant to the patient's anatomy provides feedback on positioning during the intraoperative stage. Intraoperative CAS technology supports the accurate positioning of the PSI, which is a prerequisite for achieving the intended treatment effect of the personalized implant. In light of this symbiosis, surgical reconstruction with a PSI can be considered the pinnacle of both CAS and personalized medicine in orbital reconstruction.

Several larger comparative studies have demonstrated the beneficial effects of (components of) CAS on the accuracy of volumetric reconstruction [62], clinical outcome [36], and need for revision surgery [63]. In practice, a combination of several CAS building stones is often utilized. This yields heterogeneity in surgical approaches, which makes it difficult to compare outcomes between studies. Differences in indication, patient and fracture characteristics, or implant materials used further complicate comparison [64]. Isolating the effect of individual CAS techniques on patient outcome is hampered by an overlap of techniques within study populations. The individual effects of CAS techniques have been assessed in a one-to-one comparison in a cadaver series [65]. Despite limitations associated with the cadaver model and an inability to assess clinical outcome parameters, positive effects of virtual planning, intraoperative imaging, and surgical navigation on reconstruction accuracy were established.

Several indications for PSI in orbital reconstruction have been advocated, relating to defect size, location, or timing of reconstruction [22,47,49,50,66–69]. The common denominator between extensive defect size, the lack of bone support in the posterior third of the orbit, or secondary reconstruction after inadequate primary reconstruction is that the difficulty of reconstruction has been significantly increased. The possibility to perfectly tailor the shape of the implant to the patient's anatomy makes a PSI better suited for these complex reconstructions compared to implants that lack these options. Other advantages of PSIs are improved ease of use and precise, accurate fit, which leads to accurate implant positioning and a decreased surgery time [41,43,45,49,50,70–72]. Iatrogenic soft-tissue damage is prevented as much as possible since the number of try-ins necessary to correctly position the implant is reduced, and no sharp edges are present around the implant's circumference [37,72–74]. These factors lead to the high predictability of functional and aesthetic outcomes, fewer complications during or after surgery, and a lower revision rate than other implant types [37,45,54,62,67].

The list provided in Table 1 stipulates an ever-increasing armamentarium of design features to improve (ease of) positioning or alleviate clinical symptoms. The positioning-related characteristics guarantee adequate implant support and a unique, compelling fit for the implant. It is vital to evaluate the surgical accuracy of the PSI reconstruction and the added value of the positioning features [72]. Several studies have used a comparison between unaffected and reconstructed orbital volume or angulation between the floor and medial to measure surgical accuracy [37,75–77]. These outcome parameters may conceal incorrect implant positioning. In contrast, a direct comparison between planned and acquired implant positions will reveal all surgical errors qualitatively and quantitatively [60]. Assessing individual degrees of freedom is even feasible with this approach. The evaluation phase is an indispensable component of the CAS workflow and should be performed for each orbital reconstruction. A direct comparison between planned and acquired implant positions is advocated to maximize the potential of the evaluation phase.

Incorporating clinical considerations in the design is currently not as clear as the positioning-related features. Since the early introduction of PSI reconstruction, the overcorrection of resulting orbital volume has been suggested several times, and its use has been described (see Table 1). Still, guidelines to the amount of overcorrection are arbitrary and subjective, and not substantiated by evidence. Information about the location and shape of the overcorrection is lacking. The overcorrection may even be introduced through different pathways: it may be embedded in the PSI design or added afterwards through titanium blocks [51]. While the second option provides some freedom to the surgeon intraoperatively, the judgment is subjective and hampered by the soft-tissue reaction to the surgery (and the trauma in a primary setting). Trial and error positioning leads to the increased manipulation of orbital tissue, and any dislocation of the blocks may warrant a second procedure [78,79]. Embedding overcorrection in the design is suggested to be the best solution for achieving an optimal result [78] and could be precisely tailored to the individual patient in the future, provided the abovementioned knowledge gaps are filled.

Cost, lead time, and logistic demands are drawbacks of using a PSI [37,71,73,79]. Pricing may vary based on geography, but the process usually costs EUR 1500-6000 [57,72,80,81]. Manufacturing of the implant takes approximately 3–5 working days; this does not include sterilization, or the time needed for virtual surgical planning and design. Korn et al. described a mean communication time between the surgeon and the PSI company technician during virtual surgical planning of almost nine days for isolated wall fractures and 16 days for multi-wall fractures [82]. An adjustment to the initial design that the technician proposed was necessary in nearly three-quarters of cases, but implants from technicians with previous in-house training required fewer adjustments. Improved communication and mutual understanding are suggested to be the reasons for the efficiency improvement. Complete in-house planning and design by a dedicated, on-site technician may ameliorate planning efficiency, ultimately greatly reducing the lead time (provided the surgeon and technician are experienced and have cooperated on previous cases). In-house design is suggested to reduce costs, since commercial partners are only relied upon for fabrication [81]. These benefits of in-house design may be why surgeons who use in-house planning feel less hindered by the drawbacks of using a PSI [71].

Although this paper focuses on post-traumatic orbital reconstruction, other PSI applications relating to the orbit have also been described. In zygomatic reconstruction after trauma, ablative surgery, or congenital malformation, PSIs were found to precisely restore the anatomy without the need for additional bone grafts [83]. In secondary post-traumatic reconstruction of the orbit and zygoma, PSIs enable a one-stage surgical procedure in which the surgical order is reversed: by operating the orbit first, the functional result of the orbital reconstruction is independent of repositioning the zygomatic complex [54]. PSIs may also be used to create an artificial orbital rim and floor for globe support after maxillectomy [84,85]. The most extensive orbital PSI reconstructions have been described after the resection of a spheno-orbital meningioma or neurofibroma [55,86]. In these cases, the reconstruction of all four orbital walls with multiple PSIs enabled a predictable reconstruction of the internal orbit in the same surgical setting as the resection. The PSI design in the abovementioned cases could differ greatly from the design in the post-traumatic reconstruction of solitary orbital fractures. Still, the rationale behind using a PSI is the same: freedom of design to adapt the PSI to the patient's anatomy and a predictable and accurate final result.

4. Conclusions

An overview of the CAS workflow for post-traumatic orbital reconstruction has been presented, with an in-depth description of the techniques embedded in the workflow and a special focus on PSI. It has been demonstrated how the conventional workflow can be complemented by both CAS and personalized medicine in order to optimize the clinical outcome of post-traumatic orbital reconstruction. CAS technology has catalyzed the incorporation of personalized medicine in orbital reconstruction. The reconstruction of the orbit with a PSI can be considered the pinnacle of CAS and personalized medicine. There are no strict guidelines for the design of patient-specific implants, but several design considerations can be implemented to improve the positioning or alleviation of clinical symptoms. Because of the high predictability of aesthetic and functional outcomes, the use of PSIs has been advocated especially in difficult reconstructions. Cost, lead time, and logistical demands are known drawbacks, although they may be alleviated by in-house design.

Author Contributions: Conceptualization, J.F.S., R.S., A.G.B., L.D.; literature search, J.F.S., R.S.; visualization, J.F.S., L.D.; writing—original draft preparation, J.F.S., R.S., L.D.; writing—review and editing, H.E., A.G.B. All authors have read and agreed to the published version of the manuscript.

Funding: Funding for this research was received by KLS Martin and Brainlab AG. None of the funding parties had any involvement in the contents or decision to submit the manuscript.

Institutional Review Board Statement: Not applicable.

Informed Consent Statement: Not applicable.

Data Availability Statement: Not applicable.

Conflicts of Interest: The authors declare no conflict of interest.

References

1. Cornelius, C.P.; Probst, F.; Metzger, M.C.; Gooris, P.J.J. Anatomy of the Orbits: Skeletal Features and Some Notes on the Periorbital Lining. *Atlas Oral Maxillofac. Surg. Clin. N. Am.* **2021**, *29*, 1–18. [CrossRef] [PubMed]
2. Ellis, E. 3rd; el-Attar, A.; Moos, K.F. An analysis of 2,067 cases of zygomatico-orbital fracture. *J. Oral Maxillofac. Surg.* **1985**, *43*, 417–428. [CrossRef]
3. Hoffmann, J.; Cornelius, C.P.; Groten, M.; Pröbster, L.; Pfannenberg, C.; Schwenzer, N. Orbital reconstruction with individually copy-milled ceramic implants. *Plast. Reconstr. Surg.* **1998**, *101*, 604–612. [CrossRef] [PubMed]
4. Koornneef, L. Orbital septa: Anatomy and function. *Ophthalmology* **1979**, *86*, 876–880. [CrossRef]
5. Holmes, S. Primary Orbital Fracture Repair. *Atlas Oral Maxillofac. Surg. Clin. N. Am.* **2021**, *29*, 51–77. [CrossRef]
6. Raflo, G.T. Blow-in and blow-out fractures of the orbit: Clinical correlations and proposed mechanisms. *Ophthalmic Surg.* **1984**, *15*, 114–119.
7. Grob, S.; Yonkers, M.; Tao, J. Orbital Fracture Repair. *Semin. Plast. Surg.* **2017**, *31*, 31–39. [CrossRef]
8. Foletti, J.M.; Martinez, V.; Haen, P.; Godio-Raboutet, Y.; Guyot, L.; Thollon, L. Finite element analysis of the human orbit. Behavior of titanium mesh for orbital floor reconstruction in case of trauma recurrence. *J. Stomatol. Oral Maxillofac. Surg.* **2019**, *120*, 91–94. [CrossRef]
9. Dubois, L.; Dillon, J.; Jansen, J.; Becking, A.G. Ongoing Debate in Clinical Decision Making in Orbital Fractures: Indications, Timing, and Biomaterials. *Atlas Oral Maxillofac. Surg. Clin. N. Am.* **2021**, *29*, 29–39. [CrossRef]
10. Wevers, M.; Strabbing, E.M.; Engin, O.; Gardeniers, M.; Koudstaal, M.J. CT parameters in pure orbital wall fractures and their relevance in the choice of treatment and patient outcome: A systematic review. *Int. J. Oral Maxillofac. Surg.* **2022**, *51*, 782–789. [CrossRef]
11. Choi, A.; Sisson, A.; Olson, K.; Sivam, S. Predictors of Delayed Enophthalmos After Orbital Fractures: A Systematic Review. *Facial Plast. Surg. Aesthet. Med.* **2022**. [CrossRef] [PubMed]
12. Burnstine, M.A. Clinical recommendations for repair of isolated orbital floor fractures: An evidence-based analysis. *Ophthalmology* **2002**, *109*, 1207–1210. [CrossRef]
13. Jansen, J.; Dubois, L.; Maal, T.J.J.; Mourits, M.P.; Jellema, H.M.; Neomagus, P.; de Lange, J.; Hartman, L.J.C.; Gooris, P.J.J.; Becking, A.G. A nonsurgical approach with repeated orthoptic evaluation is justified for most blow-out fractures. *J. Craniomaxillofac. Surg.* **2020**, *48*, 560–568. [CrossRef]
14. Dubois, L.; Steenen, S.A.; Gooris, P.J.; Mourits, M.P.; Becking, A.G. Controversies in orbital reconstruction–I. Defect-driven orbital reconstruction: A systematic review. *Int. J. Oral Maxillofac. Surg.* **2015**, *44*, 308–315. [CrossRef]
15. Dubois, L.; Steenen, S.A.; Gooris, P.J.; Bos, R.R.; Becking, A.G. Controversies in orbital reconstruction-III. Biomaterials for orbital reconstruction: A review with clinical recommendations. *Int. J. Oral Maxillofac. Surg.* **2016**, *45*, 41–50. [CrossRef] [PubMed]
16. Metzger, M.C.; Schön, R.; Tetzlaf, R.; Weyer, N.; Rafii, A.; Gellrich, N.C.; Schmelzeisen, R. Topographical CT-data analysis of the human orbital floor. *Int. J. Oral Maxillofac. Surg.* **2007**, *36*, 45–53. [CrossRef] [PubMed]
17. Cornelius, C.P.; Mayer, P.; Ehrenfeld, M.; Metzger, M.C. The orbits–anatomical features in view of innovative surgical methods. *Facial Plast. Surg.* **2014**, *30*, 487–508. [CrossRef]
18. Gooris, P.J.J.; Muller, B.S.; Dubois, L.; Bergsma, J.E.; Mensink, G.; van den Ham, M.F.E.; Becking, A.G.; Seubring, K. Finding the Ledge: Sagittal Analysis of Bony Landmarks of the Orbit. *J. Oral Maxillofac. Surg.* **2017**, *75*, 2613–2627. [CrossRef]
19. Schlittler, F.; Schmidli, A.; Wagner, F.; Michel, C.; Mottini, M.; Lieger, O. What Is the Incidence of Implant Malpositioning and Revision Surgery After Orbital Repair? *J. Oral Maxillofac. Surg.* **2018**, *76*, 146–153. [CrossRef]
20. Chung, S.Y.; Langer, P.D. Pediatric orbital blowout fractures. *Curr. Opin. Ophthalmol.* **2017**, *28*, 470–476. [CrossRef]
21. Schreurs, R.; Wilde, F.; Schramm, A.; Gellrich, N.C. Intraoperative Feedback and Quality Control in Orbital Reconstruction: The Past, the Present, and the Future. *Atlas Oral Maxillofac. Surg. Clin. N. Am.* **2021**, *29*, 97–108. [CrossRef] [PubMed]
22. Schreurs, R.; Klop, C.; Gooris, P.J.J.; Maal, T.J.J.; Becking, A.G.; Dubois, L. Critical appraisal of patient-specific implants for secondary post-traumatic orbital reconstruction. *Int. J. Oral Maxillofac. Surg.* **2022**, *51*, 790–798. [CrossRef] [PubMed]
23. Nkenke, E.; Maier, T.; Benz, M.; Wiltfang, J.; Holbach, L.M.; Kramer, M.; Häusler, G.; Neukam, F.W. Hertel exophthalmometry versus computed tomography and optical 3D imaging for the determination of the globe position in zygomatic fractures. *Int. J. Oral Maxillofac. Surg.* **2004**, *33*, 125–133. [CrossRef]
24. Davanger, M. Principles and sources of error in exophthalmometry. A new exophthalmometer. *Acta Ophthalmol.* **1970**, *48*, 625–633.
25. Traber, G.; Kordic, H.; Knecht, P.; Chaloupka, K. Hypoglobus—Illusive or real? Etiologies of vertical globe displacement in a tertiary referral centre. *Klinische Monatsblatter Augenheilkunde* **2013**, *230*, 376–379. [CrossRef] [PubMed]

26. Gart, M.S.; Gosain, A.K. Evidence-Based Medicine: Orbital Floor Fractures. *Plast. Reconstr. Surg.* **2014**, *134*, 1345–1355. [CrossRef] [PubMed]
27. Willaert, R.; Shaheen, E.; Deferm, J.; Vermeersch, H.; Jacobs, R.; Mombaerts, I. Three-dimensional characterisation of the globe position in the orbit. *Graefes Arch. Clin. Exp. Ophthalmol.* **2020**, *258*, 1527–1532. [CrossRef]
28. Braaksma-Besselink, Y.; Jellema, H.M. Orthoptic Evaluation and Treatment in Orbital Fractures. *Atlas Oral Maxillofac. Surg. Clin. N. Am.* **2021**, *29*, 41–50. [CrossRef]
29. Matic, D.B.; Tse, R.; Banerjee, A.; Moore, C.C. Rounding of the inferior rectus muscle as a predictor of enophthalmos in orbital floor fractures. *J. Craniofac. Surg.* **2007**, *18*, 127–132. [CrossRef]
30. Banerjee, A.; Moore, C.C.; Tse, R.; Matic, D. Rounding of the inferior rectus muscle as an indication of orbital floor fracture with periorbital disruption. *J. Otolaryngol.* **2007**, *36*, 175–180. [CrossRef]
31. Kang, S.J.; Lee, K.A.; Sun, H. Swelling of the inferior rectus muscle and enophthalmos in orbital floor fracture. *J. Craniofac. Surg.* **2013**, *24*, 687–688. [CrossRef] [PubMed]
32. Freund, M.; Hähnel, S.; Sartor, K. The value of magnetic resonance imaging in the diagnosis of orbital floor fractures. *Eur. Radiol.* **2002**, *12*, 1127–1133. [CrossRef] [PubMed]
33. Jansen, J.; Dubois, L.; Schreurs, R.; Gooris, P.J.J.; Maal, T.J.J.; Beenen, L.F.; Becking, A.G. Should Virtual Mirroring Be Used in the Preoperative Planning of an Orbital Reconstruction? *J. Oral Maxillofac. Surg.* **2018**, *76*, 380–387. [CrossRef] [PubMed]
34. Regensburg, N.I.; Kok, P.H.; Zonneveld, F.W.; Baldeschi, L.; Saeed, P.; Wiersinga, W.M.; Mourits, M.P. A new and validated CT-based method for the calculation of orbital soft tissue volumes. *Investig. Ophthalmol. Vis. Sci.* **2008**, *49*, 1758–1762. [CrossRef]
35. Jansen, J.; Schreurs, R.; Dubois, L.; Maal, T.J.J.; Gooris, P.J.J.; Becking, A.G. The advantages of advanced computer-assisted diagnostics and three-dimensional preoperative planning on implant position in orbital reconstruction. *J. Craniomaxillofac. Surg.* **2018**, *46*, 715–721. [CrossRef]
36. Cai, E.Z.; Koh, Y.P.; Hing, E.C.; Low, J.R.; Shen, J.Y.; Wong, H.C.; Sundar, G.; Lim, T.C. Computer-assisted navigational surgery improves outcomes in orbital reconstructive surgery. *J. Craniofac. Surg.* **2012**, *23*, 1567–1573. [CrossRef]
37. Rana, M.; Chui, C.H.K.; Wagner, M.; Zimmerer, R.; Rana, M.; Gellrich, N.-C. Increasing the Accuracy of Orbital Reconstruction With Selective Laser-Melted Patient-Specific Implants Combined With Intraoperative Navigation. *J. Oral Maxillofac. Surg.* **2015**, *73*, 1113–1118. [CrossRef]
38. Kärkkäinen, M.; Wilkman, T.; Mesimäki, K.; Snäll, J. Primary reconstruction of orbital fractures using patient-specific titanium milled implants: The Helsinki protocol. *Br. J. Oral Maxillofac. Surg.* **2018**, *56*, 791–796. [CrossRef]
39. Gander, T.; Essig, H.; Metzler, P.; Lindhorst, D.; Dubois, L.; Rücker, M.; Schumann, P. Patient specific implants (PSI) in reconstruction of orbital floor and wall fractures. *J. Craniomaxillofac. Surg.* **2015**, *43*, 126–130. [CrossRef]
40. Gellrich, N.C.; Dittmann, J.; Spalthoff, S.; Jehn, P.; Tavassol, F.; Zimmerer, R. Current Strategies in Post-traumatic Orbital Reconstruction. *J. Maxillofac. Oral Surg.* **2019**, *18*, 483–489. [CrossRef]
41. Blumer, M.; Essig, H.; Steigmiller, K.; Wagner, M.E.; Gander, T. Surgical Outcomes of Orbital Fracture Reconstruction Using Patient-Specific Implants. *J. Oral Maxillofac. Surg.* **2021**, *79*, 1302–1312. [CrossRef] [PubMed]
42. Hajibandeh, J.; Be, A.; Lee, C. Custom Interlocking Implants for Primary and Secondary Reconstruction of Large Orbital Floor Defects: Case Series and Description of Workflow. *J. Oral Maxillofac. Surg.* **2021**, *79*, 2539.e1–2539.e10. [CrossRef] [PubMed]
43. Zeller, A.N.; Neuhaus, M.T.; Gessler, N.; Skade, S.; Korn, P.; Jehn, P.; Gellrich, N.C.; Zimmerer, R.M. Self-centering second-generation patient-specific functionalized implants for deep orbital reconstruction. *J. Stomatol. Oral Maxillofac. Surg.* **2021**, *122*, 372–380. [CrossRef] [PubMed]
44. Kormi, E.; Männistö, V.; Lusila, N.; Naukkarinen, H.; Suojanen, J. Accuracy of Patient-Specific Meshes as a Reconstruction of Orbital Floor Blow-Out Fractures. *J. Craniofac. Surg.* **2021**, *32*, e116–e119. [CrossRef]
45. Bachelet, J.T.; Cordier, G.; Porcheray, M.; Bourlet, J.; Gleizal, A.; Foletti, J.M. Orbital Reconstruction by Patient-Specific Implant Printed in Porous Titanium: A Retrospective Case Series of 12 Patients. *J. Oral Maxillofac. Surg.* **2018**, *76*, 2161–2167. [CrossRef]
46. Mommaerts, M.Y.; Büttner, M.; Vercruysse, H., Jr.; Wauters, L.; Beerens, M. Orbital Wall Reconstruction with Two-Piece Puzzle 3D Printed Implants: Technical Note. *Craniomaxillofac. Trauma Reconstr.* **2016**, *9*, 55–61. [CrossRef]
47. Holmes, S.; Schlittler, F.L. Going beyond the limitations of the non-patient-specific implant in titanium reconstruction of the orbit. *Br. J. Oral Maxillofac. Surg.* **2021**, *59*, 1074–1078. [CrossRef]
48. Tikkanen, J.; Mesimäki, K.; Snäll, J. Patient-specific two-piece screwless implant for the reconstruction of a large orbital fracture. *Br. J. Oral Maxillofac. Surg.* **2020**, *58*, 112–113. [CrossRef]
49. Baumann, A.; Sinko, K.; Dorner, G. Late Reconstruction of the Orbit With Patient-Specific Implants Using Computer-Aided Planning and Navigation. *J. Oral Maxillofac. Surg.* **2015**, *73*, S101–S106. [CrossRef]
50. Pedemonte Trewhela, C.; Díaz Reiher, M.; Muñoz Zavala, T.; González Mora, L.E.; Vargas Farren, I. Correction of Delayed Traumatic Enophthalmos Using Customized Orbital Implants. *J. Oral Maxillofac. Surg.* **2018**, *76*, 1937–1945. [CrossRef]
51. Spalthoff, S.; Dittmann, J.; Zimmerer, R.; Jehn, P.; Tavassol, F.; Gellrich, N.C. Intraorbital volume augmentation with patient-specific titanium spacers. *J. Stomatol. Oral Maxillofac. Surg.* **2020**, *121*, 133–139. [CrossRef] [PubMed]
52. Dubois, L.; Essig, H.; Schreurs, R.; Jansen, J.; Maal, T.J.; Gooris, P.J.; Becking, A.G. Predictability in orbital reconstruction. A human cadaver study, part III: Implant-oriented navigation for optimized reconstruction. *J. Craniomaxillofac. Surg.* **2015**, *43*, 2050–2056. [CrossRef] [PubMed]

53. Kittichokechai, P.; Sirichatchai, K.; Puncreobutr, C.; Lohwongwatana, B.; Saonanon, P. A Novel Patient-specific Titanium Mesh Implant Design for Reconstruction of Complex Orbital Fracture. *Plast. Reconstr. Surg. Glob. Open* **2022**, *10*, e4081. [CrossRef] [PubMed]
54. Schreurs, R.; Dubois, L.; Becking, A.G.; Maal, T.J.J. The orbit first! A novel surgical treatment protocol for secondary orbitozygomatic reconstruction. *J. Craniomaxillofac. Surg.* **2017**, *45*, 1043–1050. [CrossRef]
55. Sabelis, J.F.; Youssef, S.; Hoefnagels, F.W.A.; Becking, A.G.; Schreurs, R.; Dubois, L. Technical Note on Three- and Four-Wall Orbital Reconstructions with Patient-Specific Implants. *J. Craniofac. Surg.* **2021**, *33*, 991–996. [CrossRef]
56. Venosta, D.; Sun, Y.; Matthews, F.; Kruse, A.L.; Lanzer, M.; Gander, T.; Grätz, K.W.; Lübbers, H.T. Evaluation of two dental registration-splint techniques for surgical navigation in cranio-maxillofacial surgery. *J. Craniomaxillofac. Surg.* **2014**, *42*, 448–453. [CrossRef]
57. Kim, J.S.; Lee, B.W.; Scawn, R.L.; Korn, B.S.; Kikkawa, D.O. Secondary Orbital Reconstruction in Patients with Prior Orbital Fracture Repair. *Ophthalmic Plast. Reconstr. Surg.* **2016**, *32*, 447–451. [CrossRef]
58. Luebbers, H.T.; Messmer, P.; Obwegeser, J.A.; Zwahlen, R.A.; Kikinis, R.; Graetz, K.W.; Matthews, F. Comparison of different registration methods for surgical navigation in cranio-maxillofacial surgery. *J. Craniomaxillofac. Surg.* **2008**, *36*, 109–116. [CrossRef]
59. Schreurs, R.; Baan, F.; Klop, C.; Dubois, L.; Beenen, L.F.M.; Habets, P.; Becking, A.G.; Maal, T.J.J. Virtual splint registration for electromagnetic and optical navigation in orbital and craniofacial surgery. *Sci. Rep.* **2021**, *11*, 10406. [CrossRef]
60. Schreurs, R.; Dubois, L.; Becking, A.G.; Maal, T.J. Quantitative Assessment of Orbital Implant Position—A Proof of Concept. *PLoS ONE* **2016**, *11*, e0150162. [CrossRef]
61. Tokarz-Sawińska, E.; Lachowicz, E. Conservative management of posttraumatic diplopia. *Klinika Oczna/Acta Ophthalmologica Polonica* **2015**, *117*, 14–19. [PubMed]
62. Zimmerer, R.M.; Gellrich, N.C.; von Bülow, S.; Strong, E.B.; Ellis, E., 3rd; Wagner, M.E.H.; Sanchez Aniceto, G.; Schramm, A.; Grant, M.P.; Thiam Chye, L.; et al. Is there more to the clinical outcome in posttraumatic reconstruction of the inferior and medial orbital walls than accuracy of implant placement and implant surface contouring? A prospective multicenter study to identify predictors of clinical outcome. *J. Craniomaxillofac. Surg.* **2018**, *46*, 578–587. [CrossRef] [PubMed]
63. Nguyen, E.; Lockyer, J.; Erasmus, J.; Lim, C. Improved Outcomes of Orbital Reconstruction With Intraoperative Imaging and Rapid Prototyping. *J. Oral Maxillofac. Surg.* **2019**, *77*, 1211–1217. [CrossRef] [PubMed]
64. Kotecha, S.; Ferro, A.; Harrison, P.; Fan, K. Orbital reconstruction: A systematic review and meta-analysis evaluating the role of patient-specific implants. *Oral Maxillofac. Surg.* **2022**, 1–14. [CrossRef]
65. Schreurs, R.; Becking, A.G.; Jansen, J.; Dubois, L. Advanced Concepts of Orbital Reconstruction: A Unique Attempt to Scientifically Evaluate Individual Techniques in Reconstruction of Large Orbital Defects. *Atlas Oral Maxillofac. Surg. Clin. N. Am* **2021**, *29*, 151–162. [CrossRef]
66. Pedemonte, C.; Sáez, F.; Vargas, I.; González, L.E.; Canales, M.; Salazar, K. Can customized implants correct enophthalmos and delayed diplopia in post-traumatic orbital deformities? A volumetric analysis. *Int. J. Oral Maxillofac. Surg.* **2016**, *45*, 1086–1094. [CrossRef]
67. Schlittler, F.; Vig, N.; Burkhard, J.P.; Lieger, O.; Michel, C.; Holmes, S. What are the limitations of the non-patient-specific implant in titanium reconstruction of the orbit? *Br. J. Oral Maxillofac. Surg.* **2020**, *58*, e80–e85. [CrossRef]
68. Consorti, G.; Betti, E.; Catarzi, L. Customized and Navigated Primary Orbital Fracture Reconstruction: Computerized Operation Neuronavigated Surgery Orbital Recent Trauma (CONSORT) Protocol. *J. Craniofac. Surg.* **2022**, *33*, 1236–1240. [CrossRef]
69. Chen, A.J.; Chung, N.N.; Liu, C.Y.; MacIntosh, P.W.; Korn, B.S.; Kikkawa, D.O. Precision in Oculofacial Surgery: Made-To-Specification Cast-Molded Implants in Orbital Reconstruction. *Ophthalmic Plast. Reconstr. Surg.* **2020**, *36*, 268–271. [CrossRef]
70. Zieliński, R.; Malińska, M.; Kozakiewicz, M. Classical versus custom orbital wall reconstruction: Selected factors regarding surgery and hospitalization. *J. Craniomaxillofac. Surg.* **2017**, *45*, 710–715. [CrossRef]
71. Goodson, A.M.C.; Parmar, S.; Ganesh, S.; Zakai, D.; Shafi, A.; Wicks, C.; O'Connor, R.; Yeung, E.; Khalid, F.; Tahim, A.; et al. Printed titanium implants in UK craniomaxillofacial surgery. Part I: Access to digital planning and perceived scope for use in common procedures. *Br. J. Oral Maxillofac. Surg.* **2021**, *59*, 312–319. [CrossRef] [PubMed]
72. Tarsitano, A.; Badiali, G.; Pizzigallo, A.; Marchetti, C. Orbital Reconstruction: Patient-Specific Orbital Floor Reconstruction Using a Mirroring Technique and a Customized Titanium Mesh. *J. Craniofac. Surg.* **2016**, *27*, 1822–1825. [CrossRef] [PubMed]
73. Ruiters, S.; Mombaerts, I. Applications of three-dimensional printing in orbital diseases and disorders. *Curr. Opin. Ophthalmol.* **2019**, *30*, 372–379. [CrossRef] [PubMed]
74. Falkhausen, R.; Mitsimponas, K.; Adler, W.; Brand, M.; von Wilmowsky, C. Clinical outcome of patients with orbital fractures treated with patient specific CAD/CAM ceramic implants—A retrospective study. *J. Craniomaxillofac. Surg.* **2021**, *49*, 468–479. [CrossRef] [PubMed]
75. Timoshchuk, M.A.; Murnan, E.J.; Chapple, A.G.; Christensen, B.J. Do Patient-Specific Implants Decrease Complications and Increase Orbital Volume Reconstruction Accuracy in Primary Orbital Fracture Reconstruction? *J. Oral Maxillofac. Surg.* **2022**, *80*, 669–675. [CrossRef]
76. Zimmerer, R.M.; Ellis, E., 3rd; Aniceto, G.S.; Schramm, A.; Wagner, M.E.; Grant, M.P.; Cornelius, C.P.; Strong, E.B.; Rana, M.; Chye, L.T.; et al. A prospective multicenter study to compare the precision of posttraumatic internal orbital reconstruction with standard preformed and individualized orbital implants. *J. Craniomaxillofac. Surg.* **2016**, *44*, 1485–1497. [CrossRef]

77. Schönegg, D.; Wagner, M.; Schumann, P.; Essig, H.; Seifert, B.; Rücker, M.; Gander, T. Correlation between increased orbital volume and enophthalmos and diplopia in patients with fractures of the orbital floor or the medial orbital wall. *J. Craniomaxillofac. Surg.* **2018**, *46*, 1544–1549. [CrossRef]
78. Essig, H.; Wagner, M.E.H.; Blumer, M. Secondary Corrections of the Orbit: Solitary Fractures. *Atlas Oral Maxillofac. Surg. Clin. N. Am.* **2021**, *29*, 129–137. [CrossRef]
79. Maher, D.I.; Hall, A.J.; Gwini, S.; Ben Artsi, E. Patient-specific Implants for Orbital Fractures: A Systematic Review. *Ophthalmic Plast. Reconstr. Surg.* **2021**. [CrossRef]
80. Kang, S.; Kwon, J.; Ahn, C.J.; Esmaeli, B.; Kim, G.B.; Kim, N.; Sa, H.S. Generation of customized orbital implant templates using 3-dimensional printing for orbital wall reconstruction. *Eye* **2018**, *32*, 1864–1870. [CrossRef]
81. Goodson, A.M.C.; Parmar, S.; Ganesh, S.; Zakai, D.; Shafi, A.; Wicks, C.; O'Connor, R.; Yeung, E.; Khalid, F.; Tahim, A.; et al. Printed titanium implants in UK craniomaxillofacial surgery. Part II: Perceived performance (outcomes, logistics, and costs). *Br. J. Oral Maxillofac. Surg.* **2021**, *59*, 320–328. [CrossRef] [PubMed]
82. Korn, P.; Jehn, P.; Nejati-Rad, N.; Winterboer, J.; Gellrich, N.C.; Spalthoff, S. Pitfalls of Surgeon-Engineer Communication and the Effect of In-House Engineer Training During Digital Planning of Patient-Specific Implants for Orbital Reconstruction. *J. Oral Maxillofac. Surg.* **2022**, *80*, 676–681. [CrossRef] [PubMed]
83. Chepurnyi, Y.; Chernogorskyi, D.; Kopchak, A.; Petrenko, O. Clinical efficacy of peek patient-specific implants in orbital reconstruction. *J. Oral Biol. Craniofac. Res.* **2020**, *10*, 49–53. [CrossRef] [PubMed]
84. Stoor, P.; Suomalainen, A.; Lindqvist, C.; Mesimäki, K.; Danielsson, D.; Westermark, A.; Kontio, R.K. Rapid prototyped patient specific implants for reconstruction of orbital wall defects. *J. Craniomaxillofac. Surg.* **2014**, *42*, 1644–1649. [CrossRef] [PubMed]
85. Le Clerc, N.; Baudouin, R.; Carlevan, M.; Khoueir, N.; Verillaud, B.; Herman, P. 3D titanium implant for orbital reconstruction after maxillectomy. *J. Plast. Reconstr. Aesthet. Surg.* **2020**, *73*, 732–739. [CrossRef]
86. Davidson, E.H.; Khavanin, N.; Grant, M.; Kumar, A.R. Correction of Complex Neurofibromatosis Orbital and Globe Malposition Using the Orbital Box Segmentation Osteotomy With Patient-Specific Internal Orbit Reconstruction. *J. Craniofac. Surg.* **2019**, *30*, 1647–1651. [CrossRef]

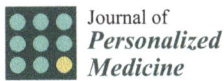

Journal of
Personalized Medicine

Article

A Contemporary Approach to Non-Invasive 3D Determination of Individual Masticatory Muscle Forces: A Proof of Concept

Bram B. J. Merema *, Jelbrich J. Sieswerda, Frederik K. L. Spijkervet, Joep Kraeima and Max J. H. Witjes

Department of Oral and Maxillofacial Surgery, University Medical Center Groningen, University of Groningen, Hanzeplein 1, 9700 RB Groningen, The Netherlands; j.j.sieswerda@gmail.com (J.J.S.); f.k.l.spijkervet@umcg.nl (F.K.L.S.); j.kraeima@umcg.nl (J.K.); m.j.h.witjes@umcg.nl (M.J.H.W.)
* Correspondence: b.j.merema@umcg.nl; Tel.: +31-503610213

Abstract: Over the past decade, the demand for three-dimensional (3D) patient-specific (PS) modelling and simulations has increased considerably; they are now widely available and generally accepted as part of patient care. However, the patient specificity of current PS designs is often limited to this patient-matched fit and lacks individual mechanical aspects, or parameters, that conform to the specific patient's needs in terms of biomechanical acceptance. Most biomechanical models of the mandible, e.g., finite element analyses (FEA), often used to design reconstructive implants or total joint replacement devices for the temporomandibular joint (TMJ), make use of a literature-based (mean) simplified muscular model of the masticatory muscles. A muscle's cross-section seems proportionally related to its maximum contractile force and can be multiplied by an intrinsic strength constant, which previously has been calculated to be a constant of 37 [N/cm^2]. Here, we propose a contemporary method to determine the patient-specific intrinsic strength value of the elevator mouth-closing muscles. The hypothesis is that patient-specific individual mandible elevator muscle forces can be approximated in a non-invasive manner. MRI muscle delineation was combined with bite force measurements and 3D-FEA to determine PS intrinsic strength values. The subject-specific intrinsic strength values were 40.6 [N/cm^2] and 25.6 [N/cm^2] for the 29- and 56-year-old subjects, respectively. Despite using a small cohort in this proof of concept study, we show that there is great variation between our subjects' individual muscular intrinsic strength. This variation, together with the difference between our individual results and those presented in the literature, emphasises the value of our patient-specific muscle modelling and intrinsic strength determination protocol to ensure accurate biomechanical analyses and simulations. Furthermore, it suggests that average muscular models may only be sufficiently accurate for biomechanical analyses at a macro-scale level. A future larger cohort study will put the patient-specific intrinsic strength values in perspective.

Keywords: 3D-VSP; CAD/CAM; FEA; finite element analysis; masticatory; muscle force; mandible; jaw; biomechanical; intrinsic strength; patient-specific; custom; bite force; muscle delineation

Citation: Merema, B.B.J.; Sieswerda, J.J.; Spijkervet, F.K.L.; Kraeima, J.; Witjes, M.J.H. A Contemporary Approach to Non-Invasive 3D Determination of Individual Masticatory Muscle Forces: A Proof of Concept. *J. Pers. Med.* **2022**, *12*, 1273. https://doi.org/10.3390/jpm12081273

Academic Editor: Peter Polverini

Received: 1 June 2022
Accepted: 27 July 2022
Published: 2 August 2022

Publisher's Note: MDPI stays neutral with regard to jurisdictional claims in published maps and institutional affiliations.

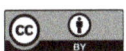

Copyright: © 2022 by the authors. Licensee MDPI, Basel, Switzerland. This article is an open access article distributed under the terms and conditions of the Creative Commons Attribution (CC BY) license (https://creativecommons.org/licenses/by/4.0/).

1. Introduction

The demand for three-dimensional (3D) patient-specific (PS) modelling and simulations has increased considerably over the past decade and is now widely available and generally accepted as a part of patient care in oral and maxillofacial surgery. Clinicians throughout the world now make use of PS modelled oral and maxillofacial implants and prostheses, e.g., reconstruction plates for oncological surgery and temporomandibular joint (TMJ) prostheses for total joint replacements (TJR). These specifically designed devices are more accurate alternatives to conventional products [1,2] and a solution for complex cases where the shelf solutions do not suffice [3]. PS designs provide a patient-matched shape to ensure a proper fit to the bony anatomy. However, the patient specificity of current PS designs is often limited to this patient-matched fit and lacks mechanical aspects related to the individual situation, or parameters, that conform to the specific patient's characteristics in terms of biomechanical demands. Most biomechanical models of the mandible, e.g., finite element analyses (FEA), often used to design reconstructive implants or TJR devices for the TMJ, make use of a literature-based (mean) simplified muscular model of the masticatory muscles [2,4–7]. This is due to the complexity of the masticatory muscle anatomy and the inability to directly measure separate muscle forces in vivo. Unfortunately, this directly affects the overall biomechanical model specificity for each patient, which is a limiting factor when the model is used to develop a PS implant that should address personalised optimisation. Relying on such literature-based non-PS muscular models when developing PS implants might result in the same mechanical failures as observed with conventional osteosynthesis materials, e.g., osteosynthesis plate failure, stress shielding, and, subsequently, screw loosening [8]. The morphology of the masticatory system is subject to wide anatomical variations [9]; thus, utilising an average muscular model is only valid for general purposes.

Due to practical and ethical limitations on in vivo force output measurements of single muscles, it remains challenging to approximate the true maximum acting forces of the masticatory muscles. The jaw elevator muscles, consisting of the masseter, temporalis, and medial pterygoid muscles, are predominantly inaccessible to measurement techniques, such as intramuscular electromyography (iEMG) and surface EMG (sEMG), that could approximate the acting forces. Both can be applied to record electrical stimuli in the muscles which, when combined with the resulting force output measurements, can be used to approximate a muscle's acting force. The iEMG technique is, however, known to cause discomfort for the subject [10] due to the needle electrodes pinching the muscle. The effect of such invasive sensors on muscular behaviour is hard to fathom, mostly because of the inability to directly measure a muscle's force in situ [11]. The sEMG technique reportedly suffers from a higher rate of crosstalk, i.e., misleading signals coming from neighbouring muscles [10,12]. Furthermore, there are many concerns regarding the sensitivity, applicability, reliability, and reproducibility of EMG measurements [10,13].

In 1846, Weber stated that the force of a muscle is related to the total cross-section of all the muscle fibres at a specified muscle length. This became known as the physiological cross-section (PCS) of a muscle [14]. It was suggested that the PCS is proportionally related to the maximum contractile force of a muscle, and thus could be multiplied by a certain constant to estimate a muscle's force. The constant is called the intrinsic strength [P] as it represents a force per unit of PCS [N/cm^2]. The resulting Formula (1) is used to calculate the muscle force (F_{muscle}) and can be described as:

$$F_{muscle} = P \cdot PCS \ [N] \tag{1}$$

Hitherto, many previous authors studied and suggested maximum values for the intrinsic strength of various muscle groups in order to determine the maximum separate muscle forces, but the intrinsic values varied widely [14–18]. Weijs and Hillen [19] reviewed the available literature on intrinsic strength and suggested a P-value of 37 [N/cm^2], based on their experimental data. However, this value was determined from PCSs measured in cadavers combined with bite force data from a group of volunteers. The intrinsic strength calculation was carried out in 2D while assuming sagittal symmetry.

The P-value of 37 [N/cm^2], determined by Weijs and Hillen [19], is still relevant as a general estimate for researchers who want a patient-specific model but only have the patient's muscle cross-sectional data available [20]. Another value frequently found in maxillofacial literature is 40 [N/cm^2] [21–24]. This value, initiated by Koolstra et al. [21] refers, however, to Weijs and Hillen's [19] value of 37 [N/cm^2].

The same relation was found using muscle cross-sectional area (CSA) [9,20,25]. The CSA, rather than the PCS of human masticatory muscles, is often used to estimate muscle force because it can be directly measured from computed tomographic (CT) or magnetic resonance imaging (MRI) data, and has been shown to correlate strongly with the total cross-sectional area of all fibres, as determined by means of dissection or PCS [9,25,26].

With this study, we aimed to propose a contemporary method to determine the patient-specific intrinsic strength value of the elevator muscles. The hypothesis is that patient-specific individual mandible elevator muscle forces can be approximated in a non-invasive manner by combining MRI muscle cross-section data, bite force measurements and 3D finite element analysis simulations, which can be used in patient-specific designs for reconstructive implants and (TMJ) total joint replacements.

2. Materials and Methods

2.1. 3D Muscular Model

Our volunteers underwent an MRI scan with a 3T MRI scanner (MAGNETOM Skyra 3T, Siemens, Erlangen, Germany) using a T1 weighed sequence (PETRA, FATSAT) and 1 [mm] slice thickness, according to our centre's regular head and neck patient oncology protocol. The subjects were scanned while in a supine position and instructed to maintain dental occlusion throughout the scan. A manual 3D segmentation of the skull and mandible was subsequently performed in the Mimics 22.0 software (Materialise, Leuven, Belgium) to function as reference geometry for further muscle delineation. Using the Brainlab 2020 software (Brainlab, München, Germany), the temporalis, medial pterygoid, masseter pars profunda, and masseter pars superficialis muscles were delineated using the brush tool. The temporalis muscles' CSAs were measured 10 mm cranially to the Frankfurt horizontal plane (FHP), in accordance with the method described by Weijs and Hillen [27].

The muscles were exported as standard tessellation language (STL) files, along with the manual segmentations of the skull and mandible. Next, the STL files were imported into the 3-Matic Medical 15.0 software (Materialise, Leuven, Belgium), where the muscles were wrapped and smoothed to obtain smooth structures. Subsequently, the muscle origins and insertions were determined as the contact area between the muscle delineations and the mandible and skull. A vector was drawn between the centres of gravity for each muscle's origin and insertion surface, indicating the muscle's acting direction. The maximum CSA was determined for each individual muscle by slicing the muscle along its defined acting direction in increments of 1 [mm] (Figure 1). The measured CSAs, in combination with the intrinsic strength values, were used to calculate the specific muscle forces. To model the muscle forces, it was necessary to assume that all muscles exert their maximum force along their determined force vectors simultaneously. A second assumption was that a single intrinsic strength value can be applied to all the simultaneously acting muscles within one subject.

The muscle delineations on MRI and the subsequent maximum muscle CSA measurements were independently performed by two individual observers (B.M. and J.S.). The inter-observer variability in cm^2 CSA was calculated in IBM SPSS statistics version 23 (IBM corp., Armonk, NY, USA). The inter-observer variability was supported by the calculating the interclass correlation coefficient (ICC), whereby a value of <0.40 is poor, 0.40–0.59 is fair, 0.60–0.74 is good, and 0.75–1.00 is excellent [28]. This statistic test is an indicator for the reproducibility of our muscle delineation and CSA determination between different observers.

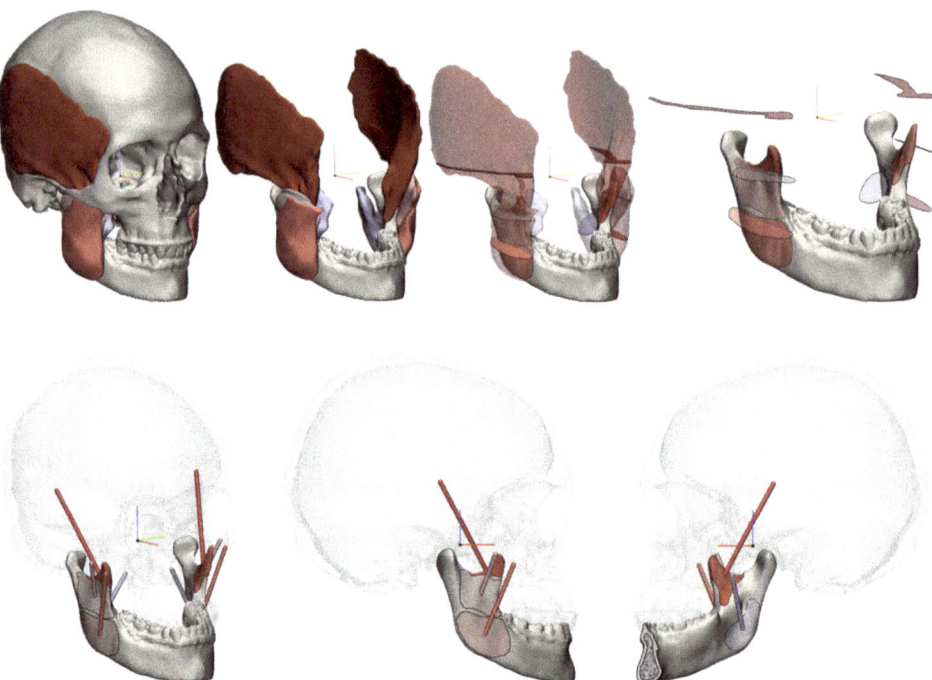

Figure 1. Visualisation of the smooth delineated muscles obtained from MRI data. The m. masseter superficialis, m. masseter profunda, m. pterygoideus medialis, and m. temporalis were taken into account. The muscles were sliced to determine the maximum CSA (**upper**), and the force vectors were calculated between the origin and matching insertion areas for each muscle (**lower**).

2.2. Bite Force Measurements

An experiment was designed to measure the total resulting force of all the elevator muscles. Intraoral scans were made of the subjects' dentitions (Trios III, 3Shape, Copenhagen, Denmark). In order to measure the maximum isometric bite force, a spacer was placed in between the subjects' central incisors to allow for a minor mouth opening of 15–20 [mm], resulting in bite sensor placement at the physiological optimum muscular length [29–31]. The intraoral scanning included both individual arches, both arches in natural maximum occlusion and the arches in a slightly open position with the spacer in situ. These scans were aligned with the MRI scan and, subsequently, the mandible was moved to match the lower dental scan of the opened position.

A bite force sensor was developed for this specific purpose (Figure 2), based on a FlexiForce A201 piezoresistive transducer or a force-sensitive resistor (Tekscan, Inc., South Boston, MA, USA). This 0.2 [mm] thick flexible sensor is 10 [mm] in diameter and its resistance reduces with increasing pressure. Using an Arduino Uno Rev3 microcontroller (Arduino, www.arduino.cc, accessed on 1 July 2021), data were collected and processed to read the applied normal compressive force. An apparatus was developed for accurate full-range calibration of the sensor. Calibration validation resulted in full-range linearity with a maximum error of 5%, measured from 30 to 560 N.

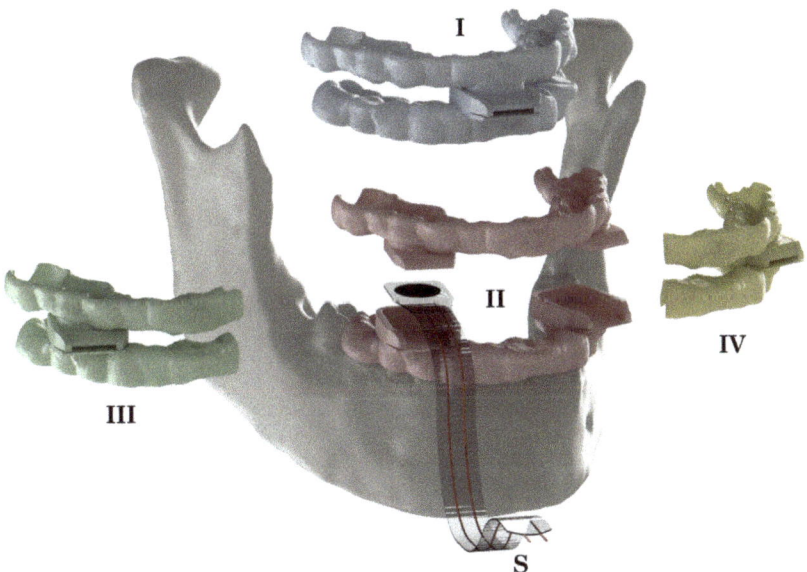

Figure 2. An overview of the used set-up including the bite sensor (**S**) and corresponding sets of upper and lower splints. The violet pair (**I**) of splints was used for incisal bite force measurements, the red pair (**II**) for bilateral premolar measurements, and the green (**III**) and yellow (**IV**) pairs for unilateral measurements of the right and left side of the premolars, respectively.

Splints were designed to fit the subject's dentition in order to prevent damaging the subject's dental elements and to distribute the bite force over multiple elements. This was performed in order to lower periodontal receptor stimulation and potential pain sensations which could influence the muscles' recruitment, and to protect the dental elements, thereby encouraging the subject to apply their maximum voluntary bite force [32,33].

The sensors were located in the incisal/midline and the first pre-molar positions since these positions are relatively easily accessible and require only minimal mouth opening in order to fit the bite sensor. The sensor pockets were positioned parallel to the FHP, resulting in a registration of the bite force magnitude in a predefined direction at predefined locations. The sensor thickness was chosen so that a mouth opening of 15–20 [mm] could be established [29–31] (Figure 1). The splints were printed from PA12 polyamide powder (Oceanz, Ede, The Netherlands).

The maximum isometric voluntary bite force was registered in an experiment that included four separate exercises, each consisting of five load repetitions. Incisal bite force was registered, as well as both the bilateral and unilateral premolar bite forces. To avoid fatigue, a one-minute pause was taken between each measurement. For each of the four bite scenarios, the maximum bite force was determined from the five repetitions. These maximum values were used for further calculations.

2.3. Finite Element Model

A 3D finite element model was set up to first determine the resulting bite forces when calculating the muscular forces from the intrinsic strength value suggested by Weijs et al. [19]. These simulations functioned as a datum measurement. In the following simulations, the problem was inversed. The in vivo bite force measurements were now used as output objective values and each subject's muscular model was scaled in output force to match these objective values and determine the patient-specific intrinsic strength value. These simulations were based on the principle of static equilibrium of forces and moments, which can be applied to an object at rest, as is the case with isometric bites.

To briefly summarise the two scenarios:

(1) Use the subject's muscle CSA and calculate the muscle forces with the intrinsic strength (P) value of 37 [N/cm], as suggested by Weijs et al. [19], and analyse the resulting bite forces.
(2) Use the subject's muscle CSA and matching measured bite forces and calculate the patient-specific intrinsic strength value.

Regarding all the scenarios described in Section 2.2, the reaction forces were measured at both condylar supports, indicating the analysed subject's specific TMJ forces and bite force location(s).

2.4. Pre-Processing/Model Preparation

The manual 3D bone segmentations of the MRI data and the intraoral scans were combined with 3D models of the skull and mandible, including the dentition, in the 3-Matic 15.0 software (Materialise, Leuven, Belgium). A cancellous volume was assigned to the mandible by means of an internal shell function, resulting in a cortical thickness of 2 mm. To ensure the correct condylar positions in our simulations, the orientation of the mandible was matched to the slightly opened position of the mandible in the intraoral scan of the dentition with the spacer in situ. The final models were imported into Solidworks 2020 (Dassault Systèmes SolidWorks Corporation, Waltham, MA, USA) and converted into non-uniform rational basis spline (NURBS) solid parts using the Geomagic for Solidworks 2021 add-in (3D systems, Rock Hill, SC, USA). All the muscle insertion surfaces were copied and assigned a surface group on the mandible model so as to distribute the force equally over the entire insertion area.

Condyle supports were used as indirectly fixed buffers to avoid over-fixation, but, at the same time, to limit the allowed condylar excursion in both the x- and y-direction of the model to allow for natural strain of the mandible. These fixtures were modelled as rectangular blocks with the condylar shape subtracted, leaving a 2 mm layer in between the condyles and the top surfaces [34]. The tops of these condylar fixtures were fixed in the x, y, and z directions and the analysed bite positions of the splints, i.e., incisal, left, and right premolar unilateral or premolar bilateral, were fixed only in the z-direction to match the bite force experiments. The contact set of cortical and cancellous portions of the mandible were considered to be bonded, and thus one part, while a non-penetrating contact set was implemented between the mandible and the condylar supports and splints. Loads were applied to the muscle insertion surfaces using the prior determined F_x, F_y, and F_z muscle force components (see Table 2 in Section 3).

Homogeneous linear elastic material properties were applied. The used Young's modulus and Poisson's ratio were $E = 14.700$ MPa, $\nu = 0.3$, and $E = 300$ MPa, $\nu = 0.3$ for the cortical and cancellous bones, respectively [35]. The articular disc properties of $E = 44.1$ MPa and $\nu = 0.4$, as presented by Tanaka et al. [36] were used for the condylar supports, while the PA12 splints were assigned $E = 1.750$ MPa and $\nu = 0.4$.

Parabolic tetrahedral solid mesh elements were used to discretise the model due to the complex anatomical shape of the mandible.

2.5. Subjects

Our workflow was applied to two male Caucasian subjects, 29 and 56 years old (y.o.), who had voluntarily undergone magnetic resonance imaging (MRI) scanning for prior research and were still available for further experiments. No subject selection was applied. Both subjects had complete and well-preserved dentitions with normal occlusions and no missing teeth apart from the third molars. None of them had clear signs of periodontal disease, pain in the temporomandibular joint or jaw muscles, or movement restrictions.

3. Results

3.1. Muscular Model

Both subjects' CSAs were measured longitudinally along each muscle's determined force vector. The largest CSAs were registered as listed in Table 1. The 29 y.o. subject's mean CSAs for the masseter superficialis, masseter profunda, pterygoideus medialis, and temporalis muscles were 4.31 [cm^2], 2.86 [cm^2], 3.37 [cm^2], and 6.92 [cm^2], respectively, whereas the 56 y.o. subject had slightly larger CSAs of 5.47 [cm^2], 2.77 [cm^2], 3.98 [cm^2], and 7.13 [cm^2], respectively.

Table 1. An overview of both subjects' measured maximum cross-sectional areas per muscle.

Muscle	Subject 1, 29 y.o.			Subject 2, 56 y.o.		
	CSA [cm^2]					
	Right	Left	Mean	Right	Left	Mean
Masseter superficialis	4.64	3.97	4.31	5.17	5.76	5.47
Masseter profunda	3.14	2.57	2.86	2.78	2.77	2.77
Pterygoideus medialis	3.34	3.40	3.37	4.02	3.93	3.98
Temporalis	7.49	6.34	6.92	6.55	7.72	7.13

The mean inter-observer variation between the corresponding muscle CSAs, delineated and measured by the two observers, was 0.73 cm^2 with an interclass correlation coefficient (two-way mixed) of 0.91, indicating an excellent match of measurements by both observers [28]. Since this study only includes measurements in two subjects, no further statistical analysis was carried out.

The direction of each muscle, as described by the vector in between the centres of gravity of the origin and insertion surfaces of each muscle, were found through the Fx, Fy, and Fz components in Table 2. The FHP functioned as the x–y plane with its positive x-axis pointing anteriorly, the positive y-axis pointing towards the left side of the mandible, and the z-axis pointing cranially. The origin of the coordinate system was set where the mid-sagittal plane coincided with the FHP.

Table 2. Both subjects' muscle force vector components for the literature-based intrinsic strength value (P = 37) and the determined patient-specific intrinsic strength values (P = 40.6 and P = 25.6).

	Muscle	Laterality	CSA [cm^2]	∑ Force [N]	P = 37 [N/cm^2] Force Components [N]			∑ Force [N]	P = 40.6 [N/cm^2] Force Components [N]		
					x	y	z		x	y	z
Subject 1, 29 y.o.	Masseter superficialis	Right	4.64	171.76	53.22	24.07	161.52	188.27	58.34	26.39	177.05
		Left	3.97	146.89	26.65	32.16	140.83	161.01	29.21	35.26	154.37
	Masseter profunda	Right	3.14	116.31	14.70	33.41	110.44	127.49	16.11	36.62	121.05
		Left	2.57	95.07	6.12	30.67	89.78	104.21	6.71	33.62	98.42
	Pterygoideus medialis	Right	3.34	123.53	7.04	57.22	109.25	135.40	7.71	62.72	119.75
		Left	3.40	125.71	11.28	61.27	109.19	137.80	12.37	67.16	119.69
	Temporalis	Right	7.49	277.18	139.94	55.13	232.82	303.83	153.40	60.43	255.20
		Left	6.34	234.64	113.21	47.02	200.07	257.20	124.10	51.54	219.30
					P = 37 [N/cm^2]				P = 25.6 [N/cm^2]		
Subject 2, 56 y.o.	Masseter superficialis	Right	5.17	191.15	57.11	33.41	179.33	126.83	37.89	22.17	118.99
		Left	5.76	213.30	67.44	49.60	196.18	141.52	44.75	32.91	130.17
	Masseter profunda	Right	2.78	102.81	17.79	31.55	96.22	68.21	11.80	20.93	63.84
		Left	2.77	102.48	14.36	39.58	93.43	67.99	9.53	26.26	61.99
	Pterygoideus medialis	Right	4.02	148.91	40.65	67.95	126.12	98.80	26.97	45.08	83.68
		Left	3.93	145.27	35.12	60.36	127.39	96.39	23.30	40.05	84.52
	Temporalis	Right	6.55	242.46	82.58	53.03	221.71	160.87	54.79	35.19	147.10
		Left	7.72	285.46	105.95	67.88	256.23	189.40	70.30	45.04	170.01

3.2. Bite Force Experiments

A total of four different bite scenarios, each including five repetitions, were recorded for each subject. All the recordings were uneventful while the subjects bit as hard as they could. Only the incisal measurements demonstrated that the subjects experienced a certain amount of insecurity or pain with the highest measured forces. The splints showed a good fit and proved to offer comfortable dental protection while guiding the subject to bite at the exact location that was used for the matching FEA. Each recording involved five repetitions of the same bite position scenario. The highest peak bite force per bite scenario was used as the maximum true in vivo bite capacity at the four specified bite locations.

All the bite forces are listed in Table 3. The $\sum$ F.Bite column in Table 3 describes the resultant bilateral bite force and is the sum of the right and left peak force in the bilateral experiment. The highest bite forces were registered in the 29 y.o. subject. The maximum incisal bite was 189 [N] while the maximum unilateral measurement was 345 [N] at the pre-molar location. This subject's highest overall bilateral bite force out of the four measurements was recorded as 474 [N] and thus considered the true maximum voluntary bite force at the premolar location. Regarding the 56 y.o. subject, we recorded 79 [N], 248 [N], and 342 [N] as the highest incisal, unilateral premolar, and bilateral premolar bite forces, respectively. In both our subjects, the registered bilateral bite forces were approximately 1.4 times (1.37 and 1.38) higher than the maximum voluntary unilateral measurements at the same premolar position.

Table 3. Bite registrations through the bite force experiments (In vivo) and finite element analyses (In silico). All the presented forces acted orthogonally to the Frankfurt horizontal plane. The boxed values were matched to determine the PS intrinsic strength values.

	Subject 1, 29 y.o.						
			Premolar Laterality			Condyle	
	Bite Position	$\sum$ F. Bite	Right	Left	Incisal	Right	Left
	In-vivo						
	Bilat. premolar	474	256	218	-	-	-
	Premolar R	318	318	-	-	-	-
	Premolar L	345	-	345	-	-	-
	Incisal	189	-	-	189	-	-
	In-silico						
P = 37 [N/cm²]	Bilat. premolar	432	241	181	-	392	330
	Premolar R	426	426	-	-	326	402
	Premolar L	425	-	425	-	482	247
	Incisal	339	-	-	339	445	370
P = 40.6 [N/cm²]	Bilat. premolar	474 (0%)	264 (+3%)	210 (−4%)	-	429	361
	Premolar R	467	467	-	-	357	440
	Premolar L	466	-	466	-	528	270
	Incisal	371	-	-	371	488	405

Table 3. Cont.

	Subject 2, 56 y.o.						
			Premolar Laterality			Condyle	
	Bite Position	∑ F.Bite	Right	Left	Incisal	Right	Left
	In-vivo						
	Bilat. premolar	**342**	195	147	-	-	-
	Premolar R	197	197	-	-	-	-
	Premolar L	248	-	248	-	-	-
	Incisal	79	-	-	79	-	-
	In-silico						
P = 37 [N/cm²]	Bilat. premolar	520	257	263	-	360	416
	Premolar R	502	502	-	-	280	515
	Premolar L	510	-	510	-	453	333
	Incisal	409	-	-	409	415	473
P = 25.6 [N/cm²]	Bilat. premolar	**342 (0%)**	168 (−14%)	174 (+18%)	-	241	276
	Premolar R	333	333	-	-	186	341
	Premolar L	338	-	338	-	301	222
	Incisal	271	-	-	271	275	314

3.3. Finite Element Analyses

The first FEAs, four scenarios for both subjects, were set up with an intrinsic strength value of $P = 37$ [N/cm²] and functioned as reference analyses for the subsequent inversed determination of the true subject-specific intrinsic strength value for each subject. The reaction forces, measured orthogonally to the FHP, are mentioned in Table 3 under "In silico", with $P = 37$ [N/cm²]. We observed that the intrinsic strength value used in these reference analyses was lower than the 29 y.o. subject's actual PS intrinsic strength, while it was too high for the 56 y.o. subject.

The results of the bilateral pre-molar measurements were summed and we considered the ultimate true bite capacity of the subject at the pre-molar location ($\sum$ F.Bite). These values were used to scale the total muscular system of the subject in the FEA. Once the right amount of scaling was achieved, the unilateral and incisal bite scenarios were analysed. The subject-specific P values were 40.6 [N/cm²] and 25.6 [N/cm²] for the 29- and 56-year-old subjects, respectively. All the post-scaling results, including the joint reaction forces of the TMJs, are presented in Table 3.

3.4. Maximum Mandibular Stress

When scaling the subjects' muscular systems, FEA showed that the stresses occurring in the mandible changed drastically for the 56 y.o. subject. Even though the location of the maximum occurring stress did not change, the $P = 37$ [N/cm²] analysis showed an increase in maximum stress compared to the calculated subject-specific intrinsic strength analyses with $P = 25.6$ [N/cm²]. The maximum von Mises stresses were found in the unilateral right premolar scenarios and occurred at the contralateral side around the mandibular oblique line. The measured values were 63.8 [MPa] for $P = 37$ [N/cm²] compared to 42.3 [MPa] in the matching $P = 25.6$ [N/cm²] scenario. Figure 3 visualises this comparison.

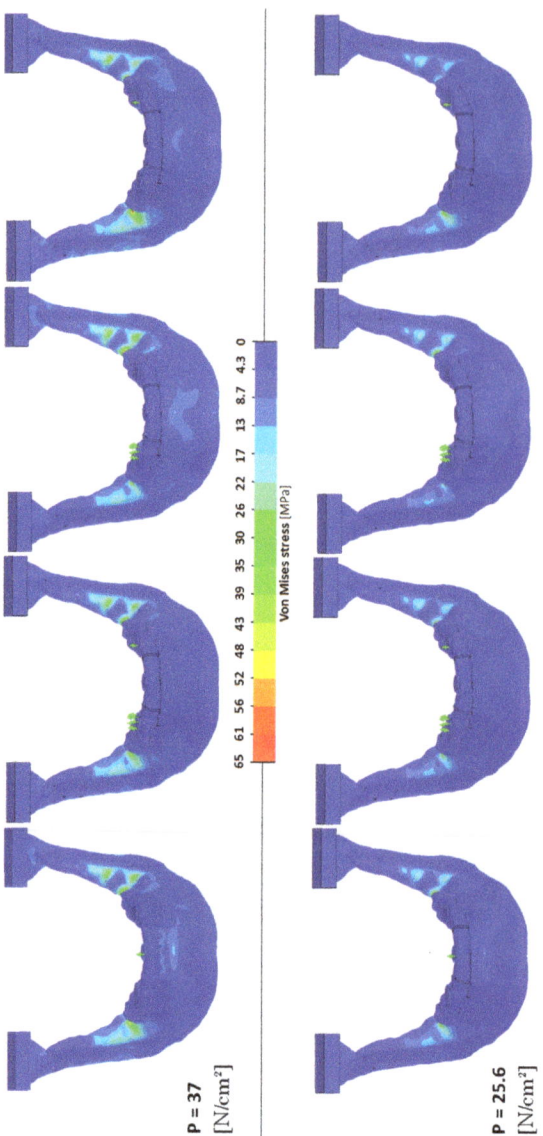

Figure 3. Visualisation of the von-Mises stress occurring in all the FEA scenarios of our 56 y.o. subject. Left to right: incisal, bilateral premolar, unilateral premolar right, and unilateral premolar left bite.

4. Discussion

We propose a contemporary method to determine the patient-specific intrinsic strength value of the elevator muscles of the mandible. Furthermore, we show how to patient-specifically approximate the value of the individual mandible elevator muscles in a non-invasive manner by combining the MRI volumetric data, bite force measurements, and 3D finite element analysis simulations.

We derived the CSAs of the elevator muscles of the mandible through an indirect 3D slicing approach. We did, however, choose to apply the single-slice measurement approach to the temporalis muscle, as suggested by Weijs and Hillen [27]. This was due to the muscle's complex fan shape, which makes it challenging to discriminate a single slice in space with the highest CSA. Our two subjects' values correlate well with the CSAs found in the literature [22,26,37,38]. Our approach of determining a CSA for both the masseter superficialis and the masseter profunda separately, instead of the masseter as a single unit, resulted in a slightly larger total CSA due to the different angles at which the CSAs were measured for both muscle sections. This separation of both muscle sections is important since it results in two different insertion areas and thus different mechanical arm lengths, which have been found to have more impact than CSA variation [39]. This effect is most pronounced in the masseter muscle, so a case can be made that dividing the remaining elevator muscles would only impact the model's accuracy marginally. Although several authors subdivided the temporal muscle into two or three sections, no clear anatomical separation could be observed between such portions, making the temporal multiple force vectors rather arbitrary in those cases [10,22]. Koolstra et al. [21], on the other hand, were successful and described a clear method on how to divide the temporal muscles into three sections.

An observation we made was the ratio between the total in vivo bilateral and unilateral bite force measurements. In both our subjects, the registered combined bilateral forces were approximately 40% (37% and 38%) higher. Several studies support this observation [33,40,41]. The majority of the available bite force measurements describe the molar bite positions. We also ran comparative analyses to determine the maximum theoretical bite forces for our subjects' molar positions using the muscular models with the patient-specific intrinsic strengths. The results from these analyses were corrected for unilateral bite using the aforementioned unilateral to bilateral ratio which should, by approximation, match the subjects' bite capacities. The FEA shows maximum corrected bite forces at the second molar position of around 365 N for the 56-year-old subject and around 613 N for the 29-year-old subject. These values lie within the range of healthy adults with natural teeth [41,42]. Bakke et al. described a normal incisal bite force of 120–240 [N] [43]. Our youngest subject's measures are within this range, whereas the measured force for the other subject appears rather low. Our subjects noted that regardless of the used splints, the incisal bite capacity was limited by a pain sensation around the teeth. According to our simulated incisal bite scenarios, based on the measured bilateral premolar bite, both our subjects should have been able to generate a higher bite force at the incisal position, as high as 271 and 371 [N] (Table 3). This suggests a biological inhibition which could be caused by signals from the receptors in the periodontal ligaments and mandible. This can inhibit muscle recruitment and thereby limit the generated bite force to prevent the anatomical structures from overloading [44]. The effect of local anaesthesia on the increase in bite force supports this thought [32,45]. We presume this has a greater effect on the incisal elements than on the (pre)molar elements due to their much smaller periodontal load-bearing surface, resulting in higher technical stress.

The current generally accepted intrinsic strength P values for the jaw elevator muscles in the literature are 37 and 40 [N/cm^2] [19,21]. In our study, we derived P values in a subject-specific manner from FEA simulations, i.e., 25.6 and 40.6 [N/cm^2] for the 56- and 29-year-old subjects, respectively. Since the MRIs were performed in maximum occlusion, our CSA measurements were performed on the corresponding muscle lengths. The bite force measurements were, however, registered at the physiologically optimum muscular length. Assuming a constant muscular volume results in an over-approximation of the CSAs, thus giving an under-approximated intrinsic strength value. Weijs and Hillen [19] observed this as well in their experiments and suggested a gross correction. If one assumes constant muscular volume between occlusion and the physiologically optimum muscular length, a change in CSA can be calculated using the measured change in muscle length. Applying a correction factor of 10% and 15%, the measured mean muscle length difference between the occlusion and slightly opened mandible positions for our subjects resulted in a corrected P-value of 27.1 and 46.6 [N/cm^2] for the 56- and 29-year-old subjects, respectively.

This can be easily overcome for future cases by providing the subjects with splints that force the physiologically optimum mandibular muscular length while performing the MRI.

Even though our determined subject-specific intrinsic strength values correspond rather well with the values found in the literature, they show a broad variation between our subjects. This variation implies the necessity to determine the patient-specific capacity of the muscular system of the mandible. Our 56 y.o. subject's mandibular stress values were 63.8 [MPa] for $P = 37$ [N/cm^2] versus 42.3 [MPa] in the corresponding $P = 25.6$ [N/cm^2] scenario. In this case, the $P = 37$ [N/cm^2] intrinsic strength, as was suggested in the literature, would have resulted in an overestimation of the muscular forces, leading to a stress increase of 51% in the analysis. Using the model to, e.g., design a PS implant or (TMJ) prosthesis, could result in a radical overestimation, i.e., too bulky or thick designs, of the final implant. Such overestimations lead to PS implants that are much stiffer than necessary which, in turn, is likely to result in stress shielding of the surrounding bone and could subsequently lead to screw loosening due to stress shielding-induced bone resorption [8]. Our 29 y.o. subject's corrected determined intrinsic strength is approximately 25% higher than that suggested in the literature. We simulated the reconstruction of a segmental defect in the mandible and found a comparable increase in the reconstruction plate's maximum occurring stress. Depending on the applied alloy and the actual maximum occurring stress value in the plate, this 25% stress increase could mean a decrease in a plate's life span of 10,000 to several million cycles [46], which would mean less than a week to several years of intensive loading [47].

We realise that following the protocol suggested by this study, as well as determining patient-specific intrinsic strength values, is time consuming and will therefore not always fit in with the scheduled treatment of a patient. Hence, future studies should aim to optimise and automate parts of the methods used in the protocol described herein. For example, the delineation of the separate muscles is rather time consuming and could be overcome by applying a (semi) auto-segmentation tool. Another suggestion would be to simplify the bite force measurements by using a commercially available tool.

The variation in determined intrinsic strength values for our subjects in the current proof of concept implies that true clinical intrinsic strength determination is complex and dependent on multiple factors instead of merely the CSA of a muscle. With the results of our small cohort, presented here, we do not suggest a new general intrinsic strength value to replace the currently accepted $P = 37$ and 40 [N/cm^2] values [19,21]. We did, however, observe the deviation between these values and the values we determined in this study, as well as the variation we found between our subjects. Therefore, it appears necessary to determine the intrinsic strength in a PS manner when critical biomechanical models or simulations are performed.

In the near future, we aim to start a study in which PS intrinsic strength determinations, as presented here, will be carried out for a large group of patients as part of the clinical evaluation. We aim to further study the spread of individual intrinsic strength values and to conclude if the intrinsic strength should indeed be calculated patient-specifically in all cases.

5. Conclusions

Despite using a small cohort in this proof of concept study, we show that there is great variation between our subjects' individual muscular intrinsic strength. This variation, together with the difference between our individual results and those presented in the literature, emphasises the value of our patient-specific muscle modelling and intrinsic strength determination protocol to ensure accurate biomechanical analyses and simulations. Furthermore, it suggests that average muscular models may only be sufficiently accurate for biomechanical analyses at a macro-scale level. A future larger cohort study will put the patient-specific intrinsic strength values in perspective.

Author Contributions: Conceptualization, B.B.J.M., J.J.S., F.K.L.S., J.K. and M.J.H.W.; methodology, B.B.J.M. and J.K.; software, F.K.L.S. and J.K.; formal analysis, B.B.J.M.; investigation, M.J.H.W.; resources, B.B.J.M.; data curation, J.J.S.; writing—original draft preparation, B.B.J.M.; writing—review and editing, J.J.S., F.K.L.S., J.K. and M.J.H.W.; supervision, F.K.L.S., J.K. and M.J.H.W.; All authors have read and agreed to the published version of the manuscript.

Funding: No funding was received for this research.

Institutional Review Board Statement: Approval for this study was obtained from the Medical Ethics Board of the University Medical Center Groningen (METc 2016/388).

Informed Consent Statement: All the subjects provided written consent.

Data Availability Statement: The authors declare that the data supporting the findings of this study are available within the paper.

Acknowledgments: We are grateful to the subjects who volunteered for this study.

Conflicts of Interest: The authors have no conflict of interest to declare.

References

1. Kraeima, J.; Merema, B.J.; Witjes, M.J.H.; Spijkervet, F.K.L. Development of a patient-specific temporomandibular joint prosthesis according to the Groningen principle through a cadaver test series. *J. Cranio-Maxillofac. Surg.* **2018**, *46*, 779–784. [CrossRef] [PubMed]
2. Merema, B.B.J.; Kraeima, J.; Visscher, S.A.H.J.; Minnen, B.; Spijkervet, F.K.L.; Schepman, K.; Witjes, M.J.H. Novel finite element-based plate design for bridging mandibular defects: Reducing mechanical failure. *Oral Dis.* **2020**, *26*, 1265–1274. [CrossRef]
3. Kraeima, J.; Glas, H.H.; Merema, B.B.J.; Vissink, A.; Spijkervet, F.K.L.; Witjes, M.J.H. Three-dimensional virtual surgical planning in the oncologic treatment of the mandible. *Oral Dis.* **2021**, *27*, 14–20. [CrossRef] [PubMed]
4. Reina, J.M.; Garcia-Aznar, J.M.; Dominguez, J.; Doblare, M. Numerical estimation of bone density and elastic constants distribution in a human mandible. *J. Biomech.* **2007**, *40*, 828–836. [CrossRef]
5. Narra, N.; Valášek, J.; Hannula, M.; Marcián, P.; Sándor, G.K.; Hyttinen, J.; Wolff, J. Finite element analysis of customized reconstruction plates for mandibular continuity defect therapy. *J. Biomech.* **2014**, *47*, 264–268. [CrossRef]
6. Pinheiro, M.; Willaert, R.; Khan, A.; Krairi, A.; Van Paepegem, W. Biomechanical evaluation of the human mandible after temporomandibular joint replacement under different biting conditions. *Sci. Rep.* **2021**, *11*, 14034. [CrossRef]
7. Oenning, A.C.; Freire, A.R.; Rossi, A.C.; Prado, F.B.; Caria, P.H.F.; Correr-Sobrinho, L.; Haiter-Neto, F. Resorptive potential of impacted mandibular third molars: 3D simulation by finite element analysis. *Clin. Oral Investig.* **2018**, *22*, 3195–3203. [CrossRef]
8. Merema, B.B.J.; Kraeima, J.; Glas, H.H.; Spijkervet, F.K.L.; Witjes, M.J.H. Patient-specific finite element models of the human mandible: Lack of consensus on current set-ups. *Oral Dis.* **2021**, *27*, 42–51. [CrossRef] [PubMed]
9. Weijs, W.A.; Hillen, B. Correlations between the cross-sectional area of the jaw muscles and craniofacial size and shape. *Am. J. Phys. Anthropol.* **1986**, *70*, 423–431. [CrossRef]
10. Abdi, A.H.; Sagl, B.; Srungarapu, V.P.; Stavness, I.; Prisman, E.; Abolmaesumi, P.; Fels, S. Characterizing Motor Control of Mastication With Soft Actor-Critic. *Front. Hum. Neurosci.* **2020**, *14*, 188. [CrossRef]
11. Wood, W.W.; Takada, K.; Hannam, A.G. The electromyographic activity of the inferior part of the human lateral pterygoid muscle during clenching and chewing. *Arch. Oral Biol.* **1986**, *31*, 245–253. [CrossRef]
12. Farina, D.; Merletti, R.; Indino, B.; Graven-Nielsen, T. Surface EMG crosstalk evaluated from experimental recordings and simulated signals. Reflections on crosstalk interpretation, quantification and reduction. *Methods Inf. Med.* **2004**, *43*, 30–35. [PubMed]
13. Vigotsky, A.D.; Halperin, I.; Lehman, G.J.; Trajano, G.S.; Vieira, T.M. Interpreting Signal Amplitudes in Surface Electromyography Studies in Sport and Rehabilitation Sciences. *Front. Physiol.* **2018**, *8*, 985. [CrossRef] [PubMed]
14. Weber, E. Muskelbewegung. In *Wagner, Handwörterbuch der Physiologie*; Bieweg: Braunschweig, Germany, 1846; pp. 1–122.
15. Nygaard, E.; Houston, M.; Suzuki, Y.; Jorgensen, K.; Saltin, B. Morphology of the brachial biceps muscle and elbow flexion in man. *Acta Physiol. Scand.* **1983**, *117*, 287–292. [CrossRef]
16. Morris, C.B. The measurement of the strength of muscle relative to the cross section. *Res. Q.* **1948**, *19*, 295–303. [CrossRef]
17. Haxton, H.A. Absolute muscle force in the ankle flexors of man. *J. Physiol.* **1944**, *103*, 267–273. [CrossRef] [PubMed]
18. Franke, F. Die Kraftkurve menschlicher Muskeln bei willkürlicher Innerration und die Frage der absoluten Muskelkraft. *Pflüg. Arch. Ges. Physiol.* **1920**, *184*, 300–323. [CrossRef]
19. Weijs, W.A.; Hillen, B. Cross-sectional areas and estimated intrinsic strength of the human jaw muscles. *Acta Morphol. Neerl. Scand.* **1985**, *23*, 267–274.
20. Toro-Ibacache, V.; Zapata Munoz, V.; O'Higgins, P. The relationship between skull morphology, masticatory muscle force and cranial skeletal deformation during biting. *Ann. Anat.* **2016**, *203*, 59–68. [CrossRef] [PubMed]
21. Koolstra, J.H.; van Eijden, T.M.G.J.; Weijs, W.A.; Naeije, M. A three-dimensional mathematical model of the human masticatory system predicting maximum possible bite forces. *J. Biomech.* **1988**, *21*, 563–576. [CrossRef]

22. Peck, C.C.; Langenbach, G.E.; Hannam, A.G. Dynamic simulation of muscle and articular properties during human wide jaw opening. *Arch. Oral Biol.* **2000**, *45*, 963–982. [CrossRef]
23. Hannam, A.G.; Stavness, I.; Lloyd, J.E.; Fels, S. A dynamic model of jaw and hyoid biomechanics during chewing. *J. Biomech.* **2008**, *41*, 1069–1076. [CrossRef] [PubMed]
24. Sagl, B.; Schmid-Schwap, M.; Piehslinger, E.; Kundi, M.; Stavness, I. A Dynamic Jaw Model With a Finite-Element Temporomandibular Joint. *Front. Physiol.* **2019**, *10*, 1156. [CrossRef] [PubMed]
25. Hannam, A.G.; Wood, W.W. Relationships between the size and spatial morphology of human masseter and medial pterygoid muscles, the craniofacial skeleton, and jaw biomechanics. *Am. J. Phys. Anthropol.* **1989**, *80*, 429–445. [CrossRef] [PubMed]
26. van Spronsen, P.H.; Weijs, W.A.; Valk, J.; Prahl-Andersen, B.; van Ginkel, F.C. A comparison of jaw muscle cross-sections of long-face and normal adults. *J. Dent. Res.* **1992**, *71*, 1279–1285. [CrossRef]
27. Weijs, W.A.; Hillen, B. Relationship between the physiological cross-section of the human jaw muscles and their cross-sectional area in computer tomograms. *Acta Anat.* **1984**, *118*, 129–138. [CrossRef] [PubMed]
28. Cicchetti, D. Guidelines, Criteria, and Rules of Thumb for Evaluating Normed and Standardized Assessment Instrument in Psychology. *Psychol. Assess.* **1994**, *6*, 284–290. [CrossRef]
29. Mackenna, B.R.; Turker, K.S. Jaw separation and maximum incising force. *J. Prosthet. Dent.* **1983**, *49*, 726–730. [CrossRef]
30. Fields, H.W.; Proffit, W.R.; Case, J.C.; Vig, K.W. Variables affecting measurements of vertical occlusal force. *J. Dent. Res.* **1986**, *65*, 135–138. [CrossRef]
31. Manns, A.; Miralles, R.; Palazzi, C. EMG, bite force, and elongation of the masseter muscle under isometric voluntary contractions and variations of vertical dimension. *J. Prosthet. Dent.* **1979**, *42*, 674–682. [CrossRef]
32. van Steenberghe, D.; de Vries, J.H. The influence of local anaesthesia and occlusal surface area on the forces developed during repetitive maximal clenching efforts. *J. Periodontal. Res.* **1978**, *13*, 270–274. [CrossRef] [PubMed]
33. van der Bilt, A.; Tekamp, A.; van der Glas, H.; Abbink, J. Bite force and electromyograpy during maximum unilateral and bilateral clenching. *Eur. J. Oral Sci.* **2008**, *116*, 217–222. [CrossRef] [PubMed]
34. Samii, M.; Draf, W.; Lang, J. *Surgery of the Skull Base*; Springer: Berlin/Heidelberg, Germany, 1989; pp. 41–42. [CrossRef]
35. Ramos, A.; Mesnard, M. A new condyle implant design concept for an alloplastic temporomandibular joint in bone resorption cases. *J. Cranio-Maxillofac. Surg.* **2016**, *44*, 1670–1677. [CrossRef] [PubMed]
36. Tanaka, E.; del Pozo, R.; Tanaka, M.; Asai, D.; Hirose, M.; Iwabe, T.; Tanne, K. Three-dimensional finite element analysis of human temporomandibular joint with and without disc displacement during jaw opening. *Med. Eng. Phys.* **2004**, *26*, 503–511. [CrossRef] [PubMed]
37. Toro-Ibacache, V.; Zapata MuNoz, V.; O'Higgins, P. The Predictability from Skull Morphology of Temporalis and Masseter Muscle Cross-Sectional Areas in Humans. *Anat. Rec.* **2015**, *298*, 1261–1270. [CrossRef]
38. Langenbach, G.E.; Hannam, A.G. The role of passive muscle tensions in a three-dimensional dynamic model of the human jaw. *Arch. Oral Biol.* **1999**, *44*, 557–573. [CrossRef]
39. Koolstra, J.H.; van Eijden, T.M.G.J.; Weijs, W.A. Three-Dimensional performance of the human masticatory system: The influence of the orientation and physiological cross-section of the masticatory muscles. In *International Series on Biomechanics 7-A*; Free University Press: Amsterdam, The Netherlands, 1988; pp. 101–106.
40. Tortopidis, D.; Lyons, M.F.; Baxendale, R.H.; Gilmour, W.H. The variability of bite force measurement between sessions, in different positions within the dental arch. *J. Oral Rehabil.* **1998**, *25*, 681–686. [CrossRef]
41. Bakke, M.; Michler, L.; Han, K.; Moller, E. Clinical significance of isometric bite force versus electrical activity in temporal and masseter muscles. *Scand. J. Dent. Res.* **1989**, *97*, 539–551. [CrossRef]
42. Hagberg, C. Assessment of bite force: A review. *J. Cranio-Maxillofac. Disord.* **1987**, *1*, 162–169.
43. Bakke, M. Mandibular elevator muscles: Physiology, action, and effect of dental occlusion. *Scand. J. Dent. Res.* **1993**, *101*, 314–331. [CrossRef]
44. van Loon, J.P.; Otten, E.; Falkenstrom, C.H.; de Bont, L.G.; Verkerke, G.J. Loading of a unilateral temporomandibular joint prosthesis: A three-dimensional mathematical study. *J. Dent. Res.* **1998**, *77*, 1939–1947. [CrossRef] [PubMed]
45. Orchardson, R.; MacFarlane, S.H. The effect of local periodontal anaesthesia on the maximum biting force achieved by human subjects. *Arch. Oral Biol.* **1980**, *25*, 799–804. [CrossRef]
46. Fintova, S.; Dlhý, P.; Mertová, K.; Chlup, Z.; Duchek, M.; Procházka, R.; Hutař, P. Fatigue properties of UFG Ti grade 2 dental implant vs. conventionally tested smooth specimens. *J. Mech. Behav. Biomed. Mater.* **2021**, *123*, 104715. [CrossRef] [PubMed]
47. van Loon, J.P.; Verkerke, G.J.; de Vries, M.P.; de Bont, L.G. Design and wear testing of a temporomandibular joint prosthesis articulation. *J. Dent. Res.* **2000**, *79*, 715–721. [CrossRef] [PubMed]

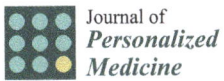

Article

Quantitative Three-Dimensional Computed Tomography Measurements Provide a Precise Diagnosis of Fractures of the Mandibular Condylar Process

Enkh-Orchlon Batbayar [1,*], Nick Assink [2,3], Joep Kraeima [3,4], Anne M. L. Meesters [2,3], Ruud R. M. Bos [4], Arjan Vissink [4], Max J. H. Witjes [3,4] and Baucke van Minnen [4,*]

1. Department of Oral and Maxillofacial Surgery, School of Dentistry, Mongolian National University of Medical Sciences, Zorig Street, Ulaanbaatar 14210, Mongolia
2. Department of Surgery, University Medical Center Groningen, University of Groningen, 9713 GZ Groningen, The Netherlands; n.assink@umcg.nl (N.A.); a.m.l.meesters@umcg.nl (A.M.L.M.)
3. 3D Lab, University Medical Center Groningen, University of Groningen, 9713 GZ Groningen, The Netherlands; j.kraeima@umcg.nl (J.K.); m.j.h.witjes@umcg.nl (M.J.H.W.)
4. Department of Oral and Maxillofacial Surgery, University Medical Center Groningen, University of Groningen, 9713 GZ Groningen, The Netherlands; r.r.m.bos@umcg.nl (R.R.M.B.); a.vissink@umcg.nl (A.V.)
* Correspondence: enkhorchlon@mnums.edu.mn (E.-O.B.); b.van.minnen@umcg.nl (B.v.M.)

Abstract: As 2D quantitative measurements are often insufficient, a standardized 3D quantitative measurement method was developed to analyze mandibular condylar fractures, and correlate the results with the mandibular condylar fracture classifications of Loukota and Spiessl and Schroll and clinical parameters. Thirty-two patients with a unilateral mandibular condylar fracture were evaluated using OPT, 2D (CB)CT images, and 3D imaging to measure the extent of the fractures. The maximum mouth opening (MMO) was measured. Ramus height loss could be measured only in OPT, but not in 2D CT images. The Intraclass Correlation Coefficient was excellent in the 3D measurements. In the Loukota classification, condylar neck fractures had the largest median 3D displacement and the highest rotations of the fracture fragments. The largest fracture volume was observed in base fractures. According to the Spiessl and Schroll classification, type V fractures had the largest median 3D displacement and the highest rotation in the X-axis and Z-axis. Type I fractures had the largest fracture volume. We found a moderate negative correlation between MMO and 3D displacement and rotation on Z-axis. The 2D quantitative analysis of condylar fractures is limited, imprecise, and not reproducible, while quantitative 3D measurements provide extensive, precise, objective, and reproducible information.

Keywords: mandibular fractures; mandibular condyle; three-dimensional imaging; classification; diagnoses

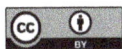

1. Introduction

Fractures of the condylar process represent 29–52% of all mandibular fractures. However, there is a lack of consensus on treatment of these fractures [1–5]. Generally speaking, practitioners chose one of two treatment modalities for condylar fractures: surgical (open) treatment or conservative (closed) treatment [4,6]. The choice of treatment modality can be based on the classification and characteristics of the fracture [4], but in practice, this choice is usually based on the training, experience, and skills of the surgeon. To overcome these differences in approach, several classification systems for condylar fractures have been proposed [7–10], of which the classifications of Loukota [11,12] and Spiessl and Schroll [13] are the most widely used.

To diagnose and classify condylar fractures, practitioners frequently use conventional two-dimensional (2D) imaging, such as panoramic radiographs (OPT) and Towne projections. Based on these radiographs, fracture characteristics such as ramus height loss and deviation of the condylar head are measured to decide on the preferred treatment modalities [14–17]. However, Kommers et al. [18] questioned the reliability of measuring the ramus height loss of fractures of the condylar process on OPT. Additionally, others showed that measurements on conventional 2D imaging are highly observer dependent and vary with patient positioning when taking X-rays [19–23].

Despite the efforts of several authors, no consensus has been reached on clinically relevant universal classification and subsequent treatment choices of condylar fractures. This situation continued even after the introduction of computed tomography (CT) [7,9,24]. Such a classification is needed because the description of condylar fractures is currently dependent on 2D slices of CT images, while the availability of conventional 2D images such as OPT and Towne is rapidly declining due to the introduction of low dose CT and the conebeam CT (CBCT) [7]. Even though CT and CBCT can display the anatomy in 3D, most CT data are still viewed in 2D slices. A major drawback of the use of 2D CT images is that the assessment of condylar fractures with this type of radiograph is also dependent on the skills of the clinician who analyses these 2D CT images and can vary depending on the CT characteristics such as resolution, slice thickness, and field of view [7]. Moreover, measurements such as the estimated loss of ramus height and deviation of the condylar head are not reliable if they are based on 2D CT images [7].

Nowadays, quantitative three-dimensional (3D) CT measurements are used for diagnosis and classification of fractures of the tibial plateau, acetabulum, and radial heads [25–28]. These measurements have been proven reliable and have provided insight into the multidirectional aspects of these fractures based on this detailed information about fracture extent [25–27]. Therefore, the aim of this study was to develop a standardized 3D quantitative measurement method for mandibular condyle fractures with high inter-user reliability, to correlate the obtained results with the Loukota [11,12] and Spiessl and Schroll [13] classifications and with clinical parameters as ramus height loss and maximum mouth opening.

2. Materials and Methods

2.1. Study Population

All consecutive patients that were diagnosed with a unilateral mandibular condylar fracture with or without concomitant other mandibular fractures at University Medical Center Groningen between 2015 and 2018 were reviewed. Patients whose diagnosis was confirmed with CBCT or CT with a maximum slice thickness of 1 mm were included. Exclusion criteria were a bilateral condylar fracture and unavailability of a diagnostic CT or CBCT scan. This study was conducted according to the guidelines of the Declaration of Helsinki. There is no file number of the medical ethical committee as it is a retrospective study that analyses anonymous CT data from our center only. The default is that this does not require a review board statement.

2.2. Fracture Classification and Clinical Parameters

To classify the condylar fractures, based on the preoperative standard 2D format CT or CBCT scans in axial, coronal, and sagittal reconstructions, the classifications according to Loukota [11,12] and Spiessl and Schroll [13] were used.

Due to the retrospective nature of this study, not all 32 eligible cases were completely documented with respect to clinical parameters. maximum mouth opening (MMO) measurements (from incisor to incisor) were available from 20 patients. These measurements consisted of MMO scores in mm on the same day (± 1 day) that the CT or CBCT scan was taken.

In patients whose OPT and/or Towne projections were taken at the same time as the CT scan (± 1 day), 2D measurements were made of ramus height loss and deviation of the fracture. Ramus height loss (2D measurement) was measured in millimeters, and deviation was measured in degrees according to the method described by Palmieri et al. [17].

2.3. Segmentation and 3D Model

Of all included patients, the CT or CBCT files were imported into the Mimics Medical software package (Version 21.0, Materialise, Leuven, Belgium) to create a 3D bone model of the skull and each part of the fractured mandible. The segmentation process was performed using a default bone threshold (Hounsfield Unit $\geq$ 226) followed by manual optimization by a trained observer (E.-O.B). All the segmented models were given a different color (Figure 1).

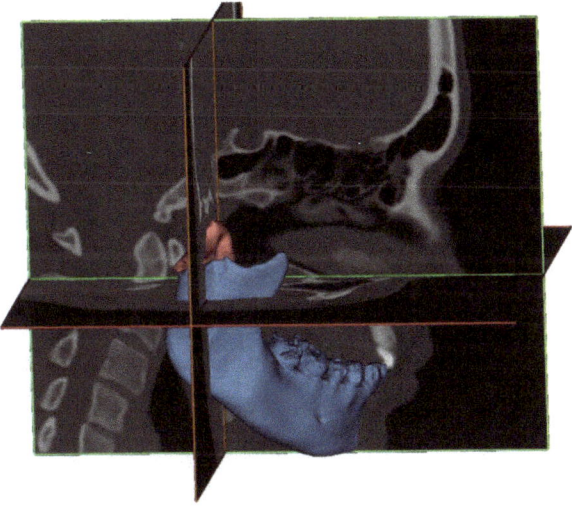

Figure 1. A 3D representation of a segmented fractured condyle (red) and mandible (blue), which is based on the CT scan, superimposed on the CT slices.

Next, the condylar fracture was virtually reduced to its anatomical position in 3-matic Medical (version 13.0; Materialise, Leuven, Belgium). As a guide for reduction, the contralateral non-fractured side was mirrored and aligned with the affected side (Figure 2).

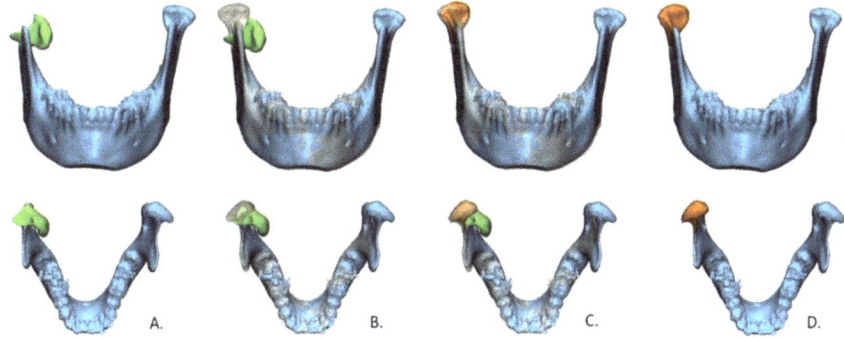

Figure 2. Workflow of virtual reduction in the fracture using a 3D model. (**A**) segmented condylar fracture fragment (green) from the mandible (blue); (**B**) template mirrored from non-fractured contralateral condyle; (**C**) fractured condyle is aligned according to the template; (**D**) virtually reduced model with the fracture fragment after reduction (orange).

2.4. The 3D Measurements

To measure the condylar fracture extent, the following new 3D measurements were used: 3D displacement, the volume of the fracture fragment and the rotation of the fracture fragment.

The 3D displacement. The 3D displacement of the fracture is the difference between the fractured and the reduced position of the condyle. This was assessed using 3-matic Medical and Matlab (R2014B, Mathworks, Natick, MA, USA) software. The extent of displacement/dislocation of the fragment(s) of the condyle was determined by calculating the 3D displacement along the X, Y, and Z axes. To calculate the 3D displacement, the fracture was virtually reduced in the 3D model, as described above (Figure 2). For each point on the surface of the 3D model, a difference in Euclidian distance between the fractured and reduced position was calculated in millimeters (mm). This 3D displacement of each part of the fragment is presented as a distance map in Figure 3, and was calculated as follows:

$$\text{3D displacement} = \frac{\sum_{i=1}^{n}(Surface_i * displacement_i)}{\sum_{i}^{n}(Surface_i) + Nondisplaced\ surface}$$

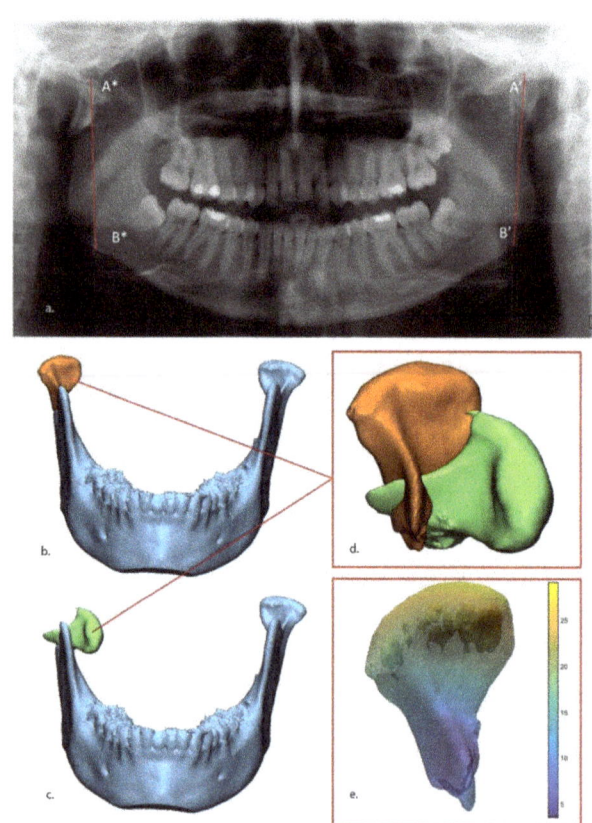

Figure 3. Measurements of ramus height loss and 3D displacement. (**a**) Ramus height loss measurement on panoramic: Loss of vertical height is the difference between non-fractured (A'–B') side and fractured side (A*–B*). The 3D displacement of fractured condyle fragment after (orange) (**b**) and before (green) (**c**) virtual reduction. The two fragments (**d**) were imported into MATLAB software, after which a quantitative map of the displacement was calculated (**e**).

2.5. Volume of Fracture Fragment

The volume of the fracture fragment is the actual size of the fractured part of the condylar process. It was calculated in cubic millimeters (mm^3) using 3-matic Medical.

The 3D rotations. The 3D rotation is a rotation of the fractured fragment of condyle in the *X*, *Y*, and *Z* axes. This was assessed using the same software (3-matic Medical and Matlab). This measurement was calculated in degrees (°). Because the orientation of the mandible within the original CT scan is greatly influenced by the positioning of the patient in the scanner, a standardized axis was defined using three landmarks on the bilateral lingulae of the mandible (Figure 4). This method has good reproducibility [29].

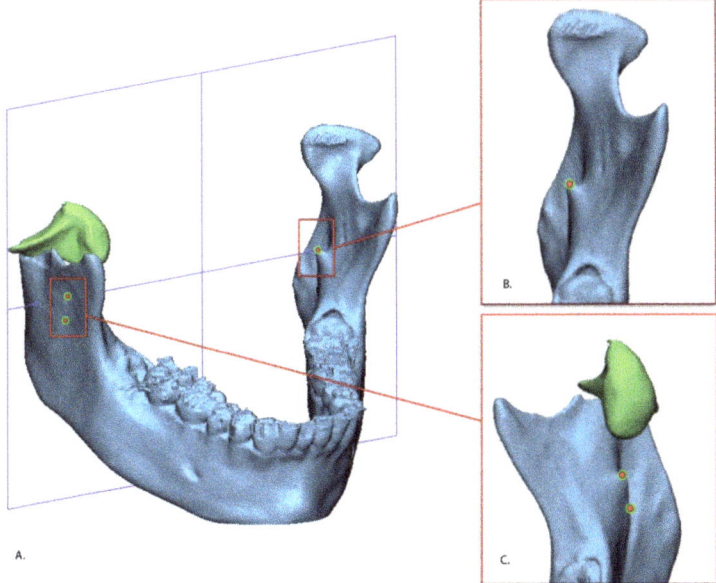

Figure 4. Defined standardized axis of the mandible (**A**). The axes was defined by using three points: The uppermost part of left lingual (**B**) and the uppermost and lowermost parts of the right lingula (**C**).

Deviation in axial alignment was described as the rotation difference along the *Y*-axis between the fragment and its original position, whereas the rotation difference along the *Y*-axis described the deviation in coronal alignment (Figure 5).

2.6. Reproducibility and Statistical Analysis

The condylar fractures were classified by two independent observers (E.-O.B and R.R.M.B.). Consensus was reached after discussion, without need of a third observer. Ramus bone height loss (2D) was measured by the same observers on the OPT.

3D displacement and 3D rotation were measured by one observer first (E.-O.B) in all 32 included patients. To assess the reproducibility, the 3D measurements were then performed by another independent observer (N.A.) in 10 patients, selected by E.-O.B, so that all types of condylar fractures were represented.

All statistical analyses were performed using IBM SPSS Statistics for Windows, Version 23.0 (Armonk, NY, USA: IBM Corp.) software. Reproducibility was calculated using the Intraclass Correlation Coefficient (ICC), with a two-way random, single-measurement model with the absolute agreement.

Normality of the data distribution was tested with the Kolmogorov–Smirnov test, and median and interquartile range (IQR) were reported for not normally distributed variables, and means and standard deviation (SD) for normally distributed variables. The

Kruskal–Wallis test was used to compare the results of the measurements (MMO, ramus height loss, and 3D) with the fracture classifications (Loukota and Spiessl and Schroll). The correlation between MMO and measurements (ramus height loss and 3D) was determined using Spearman's correlation test. Statistical significance was set at $p < 0.05$.

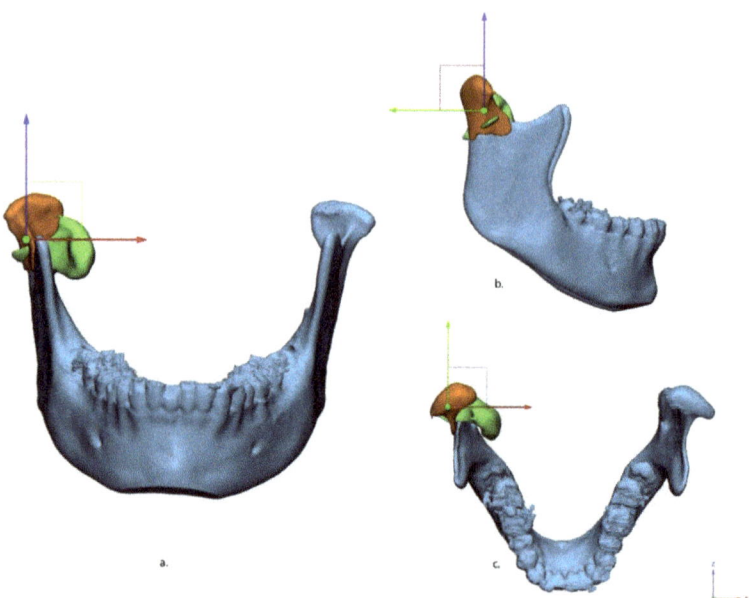

Figure 5. Fracture alignment in three views: (**a**) anterior–posterior, (**b**) medio–lateral, and (**c**) cranial–caudal. X (red), Y (green), and Z (blue) axes are shown in different colors.

3. Results

3.1. Descriptives

In total, 32 patients with unilateral condylar fractures met the inclusion criteria. Median age was 29 (21;50) years, and 23 (72%) patients were male. In total 9 patients (29%) had condyle fractures concomitant with other mandibular fractures: parasymphyseal (n = 7), body (n = 1), and angle (n = 1). The median number of fracture fragments of the condyle was 1 (1;3). The mean MMO was 22.0 ± 7.6 mm. A Towne projection was not available for any of the 32 included patients, so measurement of deviation was not possible; OPT were available for 8 patients.

According to the Loukota classification of condylar fractures, 9 patients had diacapitular fractures (type A, n = 4; type B, n = 3, type C, n = 2), 5 patients had neck fractures, and 18 patients had base fractures. According to the Spiessl and Schroll classification, 9 patients had non-displaced fractures of the condyle (type I, n = 9), 8 patients had low condylar fractures with displacement (type II, n = 8), 6 patients had low condylar fractures with dislocation (type IV, n = 6), 3 patients had high condylar fractures with dislocation (type V, n = 3), and 6 patients had intracapsular or diacapitular fractures (type VI A, n = 4; VI B, n = 2). The type III fracture was not observed in this study.

The median (IQR) of the overall 3D displacement of the condylar fractures was 5.3 mm (2.3;8.6). Median of the rotations for the fractures was: X-axis, 5.4° (−1.3;59.1); Y-axis, −0.8° (−9.2;4.5); Z-axis, 4.8° (1.1;12.0).

Eight of 32 patients had a pre-operative OPT, and ramus height loss was measured in these patients only. Median loss of height was 5.7 mm (1.6;8.2).

3.2. Reproducibility

The Intraclass Correlation Coefficient (ICC) for the validation of the Loukota classification was 0.98 (95% CI, 0.96;0.99), and of the Spiessl and Schroll classification was 0.99 (95% CI, 0.93;0.98).

The ICC for reproducibility of the ramus height loss (2D) measurement was 0.86 (95% CI, 0.45;0.97) between the two observers.

The ICC for 3D displacement measurement was 0.98 (95% CI, 0.86;0.99), and the fracture rotation measurements were X-axis 0.99 (95% CI, 0.96;0.98), Y-axis 0.96 (95% CI, 0.84;0.99), and Z-axis 0.98 (95% CI, 0.95;0.99).

3.3. Clinical Parameters by Diacapitular Fractures (Loukota Classification)

In total nine patients had diacapitular fractures of the mandibular condyle: four patients had type A fractures, three patients had type B fractures and two patients had type C fractures. Because no OPT was available, ramus height loss was could not be measured in any of the diacapitular fractures. MMO was scored higher in type A (n = 4, 24.5 mm) and type B (n = 2, 26.5 mm) fractures and lowest in type C fractures (n = 1, 9.0 mm).

3.4. The 3D Measurements by Diacapitular Fractures (Loukota Classification)

The larger 3D displacement was measured in (n = 2, 10.3 mm) type C fractures followed by type A (n = 4, 8.3 mm) and type B (n = 2, 1.3 mm) fractures. The type C diacapitular fractures had greater rotation on the X and Z axis (n = 2, 25.8°, and 13.8°) compared to type A (n = 4, 10.2°, and 7.5°) and type B (n = 2, 1.3°, and 4.1°) fractures. The mean volumes of the fracture fragments were 693 mm for type A fractures, 851 mm^3 for type B fractures and 761 mm^3 for type C fractures.

3.5. Clinical Parameters by Condylar Process Fractures (Loukota Classification)

Ramus height loss was measured only in the condylar base fractures (n = 8); and the median was 5.7 mm (16;8.2). Therefore, no comparison between the classes was performed.

MMO was documented in 21 patients with condyle fractures, consisting of diacapitular fractures (n = 7), neck fractures (n = 4), and base fractures (n = 10). Higher mean MMO was observed in the base fractures (24.1 mm) and diacapitular (22.2 mm) fractures, and lower mean MMO in the neck fractures (16.5 mm) fractures (Table 1).

Table 1. Measurements according to the Loukota classification.

Variables		Diacapitular Type A	Diacapitular Type B	Diacapitular Type C	Diacapitular Overall	Neck	Base	p Value *
MMO [mm; mean ± SD]		23.5 ± 10.9	26.5 ± 12.0	9.0	22.2 ± 10.9	16.5 ± 5.0	24.1 ± 4.9	0.235
Ramus height loss [mm; median (IQR)]		-	-	-	-	-	5.7 (1.6;8.2)	-
3D displacement [mm; median (IQR)]		8.3 (3.7;12.1)	1.3 (0.0;1.3)	10.3 (8.8;10.3)	6.1 (2.1;11.2)	10.7 (2.8;15.1)	5.0 (1.9;5.9)	0.117
Rotation [degrees; median (IQR)]	X	10.2 (2.2;15.8)	1.6 (0.0;1.6)	25.8 (19.9;25.8)	5.8 (1.1;18.1)	6.3 (1.9;35)	4.5 (2.1;4.5)	0.880
	Y	−9.8 (−10.1;−3.5)	0.9 (0.6;0.9)	−1.5 (−2.1;−1.5)	−1.5 (−9.8;0.7)	−3.6 (−17.6;18.3)	−0.1 (−1.5;7.9)	0.498
	Z	7.5 (4.8;10.8)	4.1 (2.6;4.1)	13.8 (6.8;13.8)	6.8 (4.4;10.5)	19.7 (0.4;64.6)	2.1 (0.4;9.0)	0.187
Volume [mm3; mean ± SD]		693 ± 440	851 ± 201	761 ± 72	761 ± 298	2140 ± 626	2226 ± 571	0.001

* Based on the Kruskal–Wallis test. Abbreviations: Max Mouth Opening (MMO), interquartile range (IQR), standard deviation (SD), and millimeters (mm).

3.6. The 3D Measurements of Condylar Process Fractures (Loukota Classification)

Condylar neck fractures had the largest median 3D displacement (n = 5, 10.7 mm) compared to the diacapitular (n = 9, 6.1 mm) and base fractures (n = 18, 5.0 mm) of the condyle, but a statistically significant difference was not observed between the classes.

Condylar neck fractures had the highest median rotation on all three axes; X-axis 6.3°, Y-axis −3.6° and Z-axis 19.7°. The rotation of the fracture fragments did not differ between the Loukota classes. The mean volume of the fracture fragment was as follows: diacapitular 761 mm^3, neck 2140 mm^3, and base 2226 mm^3. A significantly larger volume of the fragment was observed in base fractures compared to diacapitular and neck fractures.

3.7. Clinical Parameters According to the Spiessl and Schroll Classification

The ramus height loss was measured in following fracture types only: type I, II, and IV. High loss of ramus was measured in type IV fractures (n = 4, 8.1 mm) and type II fracture (n = 1, 6.2 mm) whereas low in the type I fractures (n = 3, 1.0 mm).

MMO was measured in 21 patients. Higher MMO was measured in type II (n = 3, 25 mm) and type IV (n = 5, 25 mm) fractures, followed by type VI A (n = 4, 24.5 mm), type I (n = 6, 23 mm), type VI B (n = 1, 18 mm), and type V (n = 2, 12 mm).

3.8. The 3D Measurements According to the Spiessl and Schroll Classification

The largest median of 3D displacement was observed in type V (n = 3, 11.9 mm) fractures followed by type VI A (n = 4, 8.3 mm), type IV (n = 6, 6.8 mm), type II (n = 8, 5.4 mm), type VI B (n = 2, 3.5 mm), and type I (n = 9, 2.3 mm). The 3D displacement differed significantly in between the fracture types.

The highest rotation on X and Z-axis was observed in the type V fractures (31.8°, 20.8°). Type IV fractures had the highest rotation on Y-axis (−13°). Fracture rotation varied in the other types of condylar fractures (Table 2). Significantly higher fracture rotations were observed in the type V fractures (X and Y-axis).

Table 2. Measurements according to the Spiessl and Schroll classification.

Variables		Type I	Type II	Type IV	Type V	Type VI A	Type VI B	p Value *
MMO [mm; mean ± SD]		23.5 ± 6.7	26.3 ± 6.1	21.4 ± 7.1	12.0 ± 4.2	23.5 ± 10.9	18.0	0.354
Ramus height loss [mm; median (IQR)]								0.143
3D displacement [mm; median (IQR)]		2.3 (1.3;4.1)	5.4 (2.0;6.2)	6.8 (4.6;11.2)	11.9 (8.8;11.9)	8.3 (3.7;12.1)	3.5 (1.3;3.5)	0.013
Rotation [degrees; median (IQR)]	X	2.4 (0.7;4.5)	4.3 (1.7;8.4)	9.4 (5.3;13.0)	31.8 (19.9;31.8)	10.2 (2.2;15.8)	1.0 (0.0;1.0)	0.021
	Y	0.1 (−2.6;1.9)	6.3 (−6.7;11.9)	−13.0 (−16.4;−2.0)	0.0 (−2.1;0.0)	−9.8 (−10.1;−3.5)	3.9 (0.6;3.9)	0.031
	Z	1.4 (0.4;3.1)	5.8 (0.3;14.6)	8.6 (0.3;−24.2)	20.8 (6.8;20.8)	7.5 (4.8;10.8)	4.8 (2.6;4.8)	0.173
Volume [mm^3; mean ±SD]		2291 ± 826	2151 ± 392	1950 ± 575	1244 ± 838	693 ± 440	793 ± 247	0.002

* Based on the Kruskal–Wallis test. Abbreviations: Max Mouth Opening (MMO), interquartile range (IQR), standard deviation (SD), and millimeters (mm).

The largest mean volume of the fracture fragment was observed in type I (2291 mm^3) and the smallest volume in VI A (693 mm^3) fractures. A significant difference was observed between the fracture types.

3.9. Correlations between Clinical Parameters and 3D Measurements

The correlations between MMO and ramus height loss and 3D measurements are shown in Table 3. A statistically significant negative correlation was observed between MMO and 3D displacement (−0.41, p = 0.05), and rotation in the Z-axis (−0.560, p = 0.01).

Table 3. Correlation between maximum mouth opening (MMO) and parameters.

Parameters		MMO	
		Spearman's Correlation Coefficient	p Value
Ramus height loss		0.57	0.23
3D displacement		−0.41	0.05 *
Rotation	X-axis	−0.27	0.23
	Y-axis	−0.54	0.82
	Z-axis	−0.56	0.01 *
Volume		−0.12	0.59

* Statistically significant results (Spearman's correlation). Abbreviations: Max Mouth Opening (MMO)

4. Discussion

The quantitative 3D CT measurement method we have described here expands the classification by Loukota and Spiessl and Schroll quantitatively. This 3D method provides precise and detailed information about fractures of the condylar process, and the reproducibility is excellent.

In a previous study, the repeatability of the 2D measurement of ramus height loss measurement was reported to be excellent using OPT [18]. In our study, however, the 2D reproducibility was good only for ramus height loss measured on OPT. This discrepancy could be related to the difficulty in finding the highest point (reference point) of the condylar head in the fractured side on an OPT in case of severely displaced and dislocated fractures (Figure 2) due to rotational movements of the fracture fragments.

Measurement was impossible on 2D reconstructed CT and CBCT images, which was previously reported by Neff et al. [7]. Our study supports this finding. Results varied depending on the slices which were chosen for the measurements. Ramus height loss can be measured on the OPT with only fair reproducibility. Moreover, this provides limited information about fracture severity. In contrast to ramus height loss measurement based on OPT images, the 3D displacement measurements of the fracture of the condylar process are precise and hardly observer dependent.

To the best of our knowledge, this study provides the first objective description of reproducible measurement of displacement and rotation of any condylar fracture. We found the largest fracture 3D displacement and rotations in the condylar neck and diacapitular fractures according to the Loukota classification, and in the dislocated high condylar and diacapitular fractures without loss of ramus height according to the Spiessl and Schroll classification (type V and type VI A). A possible explanation could be the attachment of the lateral pterygoid muscle to the condylar neck and condylar head. Although the 3D measurements are precise, objective, and reproducible, it is not known at this point whether the large 3D displacement and rotation of the condylar neck and diacapitular fractures are clinically relevant or not. To answer this question a prospective study that takes into account additional clinical variables such as lateral excursion of mandible, pain, as well as mandibular function impairment, is needed.

Limitations of this retrospective study were missing data about MMO as well as Towne projections and OPT. Within these limitations, we found a low negative correlation between MMO and 3D displacement and moderate correlation with rotation on the Z-axis. A possible interpretation is that the 3D displacement or rotation on the Z-axis, regardless of fracture classification, might be inversely related to the mouth opening. As this mouth opening was measured when the CT scans were taken, i.e., shortly after trauma, the importance of this initial mouth opening parameter to the final functional outcome is unclear.

Compared to the Spiessl and Schrol classification of condylar fractures, the classification of Loukota et al., which was proposed as an aid for making treatment decisions [12], is simplified. For example, Loukota does not take displacement, dislocation, and deviation of the fractures into account, whereas these aspects are included in the Spiessl and Schroll classification. Another consideration is that many languages do not differentiate between displacement and dislocation, which makes it difficult to translate these terms. Therefore, these two concepts must be clearly defined: dislocation means that the condyle is outside the fossa; displacement indicates the separation between the fracture fragments [6]. Based on the 3D measurements, it is possible to quantify the dislocation, displacement, and deviation in the X, Y, and Z-axes.

With regard to the validation of the Loukota classification, disagreement between the observers occurred with two condylar fractures. The first observer judged these two fractures to be a base fracture, whereas the second observer judged them to be a neck fracture of the condyle. Regarding the classification of Spiessl and Schroll, the disagreement also occurred with the same patients. The disagreement involving the first fracture was due to a discrepancy in assessing low and high condylar fractures, which was a similar problem with the Loukota classification (neck and base). The disagreement on the second fracture regarding the classification results from a discrepancy in assessing type I and type II displacement of the condylar fractures. There is no clear objective cut-off between these two types. Similar disagreement on the assessment of the condylar fracture classification was reported previously regarding neck and base fractures [30]. Together with the classification systems of Loukota and Spiessl and Schroll, the results from the quantitative 3D measurements in the present study have contributed to the objective description of condylar fractures.

The volume measurement of the fragment(s) of condylar fractures has not yet been included in any classification. This measurement not only enables visualization of the fragmentation but also provides information about the extent and inter-fragmentary stability of the fracture. It also allows an estimation of the dimensions of the osteosynthesis materials to be chosen for fixation. Although these measurements can now be performed with the 3D method, it is unclear whether this would be helpful in the clinical setting.

5. Conclusions

The quantitative 3D measurements provide precise, objective, and reproducible information about the condylar fracture with regard to volume, dislocation, and rotation of fragments, with excellent reproducibility. The quantitative 3D measurements enable surgeons to classify the fractures more exactly in accordance with the classification of Loukota and Spiessl and Schroll. Further research should be conducted with 3D quantitative measurements to determine if this method could be used to support treatment choice and, more importantly, to predict the functional outcome of condylar fractures.

Author Contributions: Conceptualization B.v.M., M.J.H.W., J.K., A.V. and E.-O.B.; investigation, E.-O.B. and A.M.L.M.; software, J.K., A.M.L.M. and N.A.; validation E.-O.B., R.R.M.B., N.A.; writing—original draft preparation, E.-O.B.; writing—review and editing, R.R.M.B., M.J.H.W., J.K., A.V. and B.v.M. All authors have read and agreed to the published version of the manuscript.

Funding: This research received no external funding.

Institutional Review Board Statement: This study was conducted according to the guidelines of the Declaration of Helsinki. There is no file number of the medical ethical committee as it is a retrospective study that analyses anonymous CT data from our center only.

Informed Consent Statement: Not applicable.

Data Availability Statement: The data presented in this study are available on request from the corresponding authors.

Conflicts of Interest: The authors declare no conflict of interest.

References

1. Iida, S.; Kogo, M.; Sugiura, T.; Mima, T.; Matsuya, T. Retrospective Analysis of 1502 Patients with Facial Fractures. *Int. J. Oral Maxillofac. Surg.* **2001**, *30*, 286–290. [CrossRef] [PubMed]
2. Jensen, T.; Jensen, J.; Nørholt, S.E.; Dahl, M.; Lenk-Hansen, L.; Svensson, P. Open Reduction and Rigid Internal Fixation of Mandibular Condylar Fractures by an Intraoral Approach: A Long-Term Follow-Up Study of 15 Patients. *J. Oral Maxillofac. Surg.* **2006**, *64*, 1771–1779. [CrossRef] [PubMed]
3. Boffano, P.; Roccia, F.; Zavattero, E.; Dediol, E.; Uglešić, V.; Kovačič, Ž.; Vesnaver, A.; Konstantinović, V.S.; Petrović, M.; Stephens, J.; et al. European Maxillofacial Trauma (EURMAT) Project: A Multicentre and Prospective Study. *J. Cranio-Maxillofac. Surg.* **2015**, *43*, 62–70. [CrossRef] [PubMed]
4. Neff, A.; Chossegros, C.; Blanc, J.L.; Champsaur, P.; Cheynet, F.; Devauchelle, B.; Eckelt, U.; Ferri, J.; Gabrielli, M.F.R.; Guyot, L.; et al. Position Paper from the IBRA Symposium on Surgery of the Head—The 2nd International Symposium for Condylar Fracture Osteosynthesis, Marseille, France 2012. *J. Cranio-Maxillofac. Surg.* **2014**, *42*, 1234–1249. [CrossRef] [PubMed]
5. Zhou, H.H.; Liu, Q.; Cheng, G.; Li, Z.B. Aetiology, Pattern and Treatment of Mandibular Condylar Fractures in 549 Patients: A 22-Year Retrospective Study. *J. Cranio-Maxillofac. Surg.* **2013**, *41*, 34–41. [CrossRef]
6. Bos, R.R.; Ward Booth, R.P.; de Bont, L.G. Mandibular Condyle Fractures: A Consensus. *Br. J. Oral Maxillofac. Surg.* **1999**, *37*, 87–89. [CrossRef]
7. Neff, A.; Cornelius, C.P.; Rasse, M.; Torre, D.D.; Audigé, L. The Comprehensive AOCMF Classification System: Condylar Process Fractures—Level 3 Tutorial. *Craniomaxillofac. Trauma Reconstr.* **2014**, *7*, S44–S58. [CrossRef]
8. He, D.; Yang, C.; Chen, M.; Zhang, X.; Qiu, Y.; Yang, X.; Li, L.; Fang, B. Traumatic Temporomandibular Joint Ankylosis: Our Classification and Treatment Experience. *J. Oral Maxillofac. Surg.* **2011**, *69*, 1600–1607. [CrossRef]
9. He, D.; Yang, C.; Chen, M.; Jiang, B.; Wang, B. Intracapsular Condylar Fracture of the Mandible: Our Classification and Open Treatment Experience. *J. Oral Maxillofac. Surg.* **2009**, *67*, 1672–1679. [CrossRef]
10. Lindahl, L. Condylar Fractures of the Mandible. *Int. J. Oral Surg.* **1977**, *6*, 12–21. [CrossRef]
11. Loukota, R.A.; Eckelt, U.; De Bont, L.; Rasse, M. Subclassification of Fractures of the Condylar Process of the Mandible. *Br. J. Oral Maxillofac. Surg.* **2005**, *43*, 72–73. [CrossRef]
12. Loukota, R.A.; Neff, A.; Rasse, M. Nomenclature/Classification of Fractures of the Mandibular Condylar Head. *Br. J. Oral Maxillofac. Surg.* **2010**, *48*, 477–478. [CrossRef]
13. Spiessl, B.; Schroll, K. Gelenkfortsatz-Und Kieferköpfchenfrakturen. In *Spezielle Frakturen-Und Luxationslehre. Band I/1: Gesichtsschädel Ed.*; Georg Thieme Verlag: Stuttgart, Germany; New York, NY, USA, 1972; pp. 136–152.
14. Bhagol, A.; Singh, V.; Kumar, I.; Verma, A. Prospective Evaluation of a New Classification System for the Management of Mandibular Subcondylar Fractures. *J. Oral Maxillofac. Surg.* **2011**, *69*, 1159–1165. [CrossRef]
15. Schneider, M.; Erasmus, F.; Gerlach, K.L.; Kuhlisch, E.; Loukota, R.A.; Rasse, M.; Schubert, J.; Terheyden, H.; Eckelt, U. Open Reduction and Internal Fixation Versus Closed Treatment and Mandibulomaxillary Fixation of Fractures of the Mandibular Condylar Process: A Randomized, Prospective, Multicenter Study With Special Evaluation of Fracture Level. *J. Oral Maxillofac. Surg.* **2008**, *66*, 2537–2544. [CrossRef]
16. Widmark, G.; Bågenholm, T.; Kahnberg, K.E.; Lindahl, L. Open Reduction of Subcondylar Fractures A Study of Functional Rehabilitation. *Int. J. Oral Maxillofac. Surg.* **1996**, *25*, 107–111. [CrossRef]
17. Palmieri, C.; Ellis, E., III; Throckmorton, G.S. Mandibular Motion after Treatment of Unilateral Condylar Process Fractures. *J. Oral Maxillofac. Surg.* **1999**, *57*, 764–775. [CrossRef]
18. Kommers, S.; Moghimi, M.; van de Ven, L.; Forouzanfar, T. Is Radiological Shortening of the Ramus a Reliable Guide to Operative Management of Unilateral Fractures of the Mandibular Condyle? *Br. J. Oral Maxillofac. Surg.* **2014**, *52*, 491–495. [CrossRef]
19. Uysal, T.; Sisman, Y.; Kurt, G.; Ramoglu, S.I. Condylar and Ramal Vertical Asymmetry in Unilateral and Bilateral Posterior Crossbite Patients and a Normal Occlusion Sample. *Am. J. Orthod. Dentofac. Orthop.* **2009**, *136*, 37–43. [CrossRef]
20. Sadat-Khonsari, R.; Fenske, C.; Behfar, L.; Bauss, O. Panoramic Radiography: Effects of Head Alignment on the Vertical Dimension of the Mandibular Ramus and Condyle Region. *Eur. J. Orthod.* **2012**, *34*, 164–169. [CrossRef]
21. Wyatt, D.L.; Farman, A.G.; Orbell, G.M.; Silveira, A.M.; Scarfe, W.C. Accuracy of Dimensional and Angular Measurements from Panoramic and Lateral Oblique Radiographs. *Dentomaxillofac. Radiol.* **1995**, *24*, 225–231. [CrossRef]
22. Xie, Q.; Soikkonen, K.; Wolf, J.; Mattila, K.; Gong, M.; Ainamo, A. Effect of Head Positioning in Panoramic Radiography on Vertical Measurements: An in Vitro Study. *Dentomaxillofac. Radiol.* **1996**, *25*, 61–66. [CrossRef]
23. Nunes, R.; Lara, Y.; Crivelaro, G. Common Positioning Errors in Panoramic Radiography: A Review. *Imaging Sci. Dent.* **2014**, *44*, 1–6. [CrossRef]
24. Zhou, Z.; Li, Z.; Ren, J.; He, M.; Huang, Y.; Tian, W.; Tang, W. Digital Diagnosis and Treatment of Mandibular Condylar Fractures Based on Extensible Neuro Imaging Archive Toolkit (XNAT). *PLoS ONE* **2018**, *13*, e0192801. [CrossRef]
25. Guitton, T.G.; Van Der Werf, H.J.; Ring, D. Quantitative Three-Dimensional Computed Tomography Measurement of Radial Head Fractures. *J. Shoulder Elb. Surg.* **2010**, *19*, 973–977. [CrossRef]
26. De Muinck Keizer, R.J.O.; Meijer, D.T.; Van Der Gronde, B.A.T.D.; Teunis, T.; Stufkens, S.A.S.; Kerkhoffs, G.M.; Goslings, J.C.; Doornberg, J.N. Articular Gap and Step-off Revisited: 3D Quantification of Operative Reduction for Posterior Malleolar Fragments. *J. Orthop. Trauma* **2016**, *30*, 670–675. [CrossRef]

27. Mellema, J.J.; Janssen, S.J.; Guitton, T.G.; Ring, D. Quantitative 3-Dimensional Computed Tomography Measurements of Coronoid Fractures. *J. Hand Surg. Am.* **2015**, *40*, 526–533. [CrossRef]
28. Meesters, A.M.L.; ten Duis, K.; Kraeima, J.; Banierink, H.; Stirler, V.M.A.; Wouters, P.C.R.; de Vries, J.P.P.M.; Witjes, M.J.H.; IJpma, F.F.A. The Accuracy of Gap and Step-off Measurements in Acetabular Fracture Treatment. *Sci. Rep.* **2021**, *11*, 18294. [CrossRef]
29. Fariña, R.; Bravo, R.; Villanueva, R.; Valladares, S.; Hinojosa, A.; Martinez, B. Measuring the Condylar Unit in Condylar Hyperplasia: From the Sigmoid Notch or from the Mandibular Lingula? *Int. J. Oral Maxillofac. Surg.* **2017**, *46*, 857–860. [CrossRef]
30. Kommers, S.C.; Boffano, P.; Forouzanfar, T. Consensus or Controversy? The Classification and Treatment Decision-Making by 491 Maxillofacial Surgeons from around the World in Three Cases of a Unilateral Mandibular Condyle Fracture. *J. Cranio-Maxillofac. Surg.* **2015**, *43*, 1952–1960. [CrossRef]

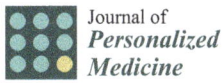

Article

Reproducibility of 2D and 3D Ramus Height Measurements in Facial Asymmetry

Nicolaas B. van Bakelen *, Jasper W. van der Graaf, Joep Kraeima and Frederik K. L. Spijkervet

Department of Oral and Maxillofacial Surgery, University Medical Center Groningen, University of Groningen, 9700 RB Groningen, The Netherlands; jasper.vandergraaf@radboudumc.nl (J.W.v.d.G.); j.kraeima@umcg.nl (J.K.); f.k.l.spijkervet@umcg.nl (F.K.L.S.)
* Correspondence: n.b.van.bakelen@umcg.nl; Tel.: +31-50-3613840

Abstract: In our clinic, the current preferred primary treatment regime for unilateral condylar hyperactivity is a proportional condylectomy in order to prevent secondary orthognathic surgery. Until recently, to determine the indicated size of reduction during surgery, we used a 'panorex-free-hand' method to measure the difference between left and right ramus heights. The problem encountered with this method was that our TMJ surgeons measured differences in the amount to resect during surgery. Other 2D and 3D method comparisons were unavailable. The aim of this study was to determine the most reproducible ramus height measuring method. Differences in left/right ramus height were measured in 32 patients using three methods: one 3D and two 2D. The inter- and intra-observer reliabilities were determined for each method. All methods showed excellent intra-observer reliability (ICC > 0.9). Excellent inter-observer reliability was also attained with the panorex-bisection method (ICC > 0.9), while the CBCT and panorex-free-hand gave good results (0.75 < ICC < 0.9). However, the lower boundary of the 95% CI (0.06–0.97) of the inter-observer reliability regarding the panorex-free-hand was poor. Therefore, we discourage the use of the panorex-free-hand method to measure ramus height differences in clinical practice. The panorex-bisection method was the most reproducible method. When planning a proportional condylectomy, we advise applying the panorex-bisection method or using an optimized 3D-measuring method.

Keywords: precision; condylar resection; unilateral condylar hyperplasia; hemimandibular hyperplasia; hemimandibular elongation; cone-beam computed tomography; panoramic radiography; imaging; 3D virtual surgical planning

1. Introduction

Unilateral condylar hyperactivity (UCH) is a growth disorder which often results in an asymmetrical presentation of the mandible. Obwegeser and Makek (1986) reported a classification system to differentiate between hemimandibular hyperplasia, hemimandibular elongation, and a hybrid form of UCH [1]. UCH is the most common growth disorder of the Temporo-Mandibular Joint (TMJ), yet the exact aetiology of UCH remains unclear [2].

The discrepancy in growth activity can be shown with Single Photon Emission Computed Tomography (SPECT). Saridin et al. described that a difference of more than 10% between both condyles can be seen as a significant growth differential between the left and right. This can possibly be used as a cut-off point to determine if surgery, i.e., a condylectomy, is needed [3].

One of the treatment options is performing a high condylectomy and orthognathic surgery concurrently. This can lead to good aesthetic and functional results [4]. Another possibility is performing a condylectomy, thus avoiding the need for secondary orthognathic surgery. In a high condylectomy, the most proximal part (at least 5 mm) of the mandibular condyle is removed surgically. This will stop further growth on the affected side, but the related remodelling of the facial asymmetry and occlusion reassurance is not predictable [5,6]. The height of the condyle removed during a proportional condylectomy depends on the asymmetry, i.e., a larger discrepancy (e.g., 8 mm) in ramus height means more (e.g., 8 mm) of the affected condyle will be removed. A proportional condylectomy significantly reduces the need for secondary surgery compared with a high condylectomy (15.8% vs. 90.9%) [7].

A recent systematic review also showed a tendency towards a proportional approach to avoid secondary corrective orthognathic surgery [8]. Hence, our clinic prefers initially performing only a proportional condylectomy on active UCH; the preoperative measurement of the ramus height difference has to be performed in an exact and reproducible way.

A great variety of measuring methods exist in the current literature to determine the vertical difference between the left and right ramus heights [9–14]. Previously, we used the conventional lateral transpharyngeal contact radiography method described by Parma [15] to determine the amount of condyle to resect. These radiographs are no longer available for daily clinical practice, so we determine the resection amount from panorex images. This is carried out 'free-hand', meaning a point is selected manually where the surgeon thinks the gonial angle (Go) is located. This point is connected to the highest point on the top of the condyle (Co). The distance in millimetres between these points is considered the ramus height. Both sides are measured, and the difference between the left and right, i.e., the amount to resect during the condylectomy, is determined. A problem encountered in our clinic with this method is that the TMJ surgeons measure different amounts to resect during surgery since this is not a validated procedure. Another commonly used measuring method for ramus height with the panorex is the 'bisection method', in which point Go is constructed by bisecting the angle between the tangent of the lower and posterior borders [11–13,16].

Unfortunately, such two-dimensional measurements on a panorex have been reported as leading to asymmetry under-diagnosis due to the angled projection of the panorex [17]. Hence, alternative planning tools need to be explored to determine the asymmetry more precisely. De Bont et al. already presented Computed Tomography (CT) in 1993 as an imaging modality to detect UCH [18]. Nolte et al. (2016) showed that measurements based on three-dimensional data, using a Cone-Beam Computed Tomography (CBCT) scan, can be used to quantify mandibular asymmetry [19]. However, the different two-dimensional panorex measurements have not been compared with each other or compared with a 3D analysis.

We asked ourselves if it would be possible to add more reproducibility, i.e., precision or reliability, to our daily practice by changing to a different measuring method. Hence, the aim of this study was to objectify the most reproducible ramus height measurement method, so that it does not matter who performs the measuring, or when. A 3D analysis method based on CBCT data was developed and compared to the panorex-free-hand method, and to the commonly used bisection method in the literature.

2. Materials and Methods

In order to evaluate the reproducibility of the 3 described measuring methods, we selected a cohort of patients who had had both panorex (Planmeca, Helsinki, Finland) and CBCT (Planmeca, Helsinki, Finland) scans within a short period of time: the pre-operative data of the patients who had undergone orthognathic surgery between 2015 and 2018 were analysed. Patients were only included if they met the following criteria:

- Older than 16 years of age;
- A panorex image where the condyle and the gonial angle are visible on both sides;
- A CBCT with a slice thickness of 0.4 mm.

The exclusion criterion was:

- Prior mandibular surgery.

2.1. Two-Dimensional Methods

Two different independent measurements of the mandibular ramus height were performed on the 2D panorex images. The first method was conducted 'free-hand', meaning the observer manually chose a point where he/she thought the gonial angle (Go) was located. This point was connected to the highest point on the top of the condyle (Co). The distance in millimetres between these points was considered the ramus height. Both sides were measured, and the difference between the left and right was determined. The second 'bisection method' (Figure 1) was based on the method described by Kjellberg et al. (1994) [13]. First, the tangent of both the mandibular ramus and the body was drawn. Another line was drawn from the intersection of these lines to the mandible, dividing the angle between the two tangents into two equal angles. The gonion, where this line crosses the curvature of the angle of the mandible, was marked. The ramus height was measured from the Go-Co on both sides, and the difference between the left and right was determined. A positive number meant the left ramus was longer compared to the right and vice versa. Both 2D measurements (bisection and free-hand method) were made for all the patients by N.B.v.B., an Oral and Maxillofacial surgeon who specialized in TMJ surgery.

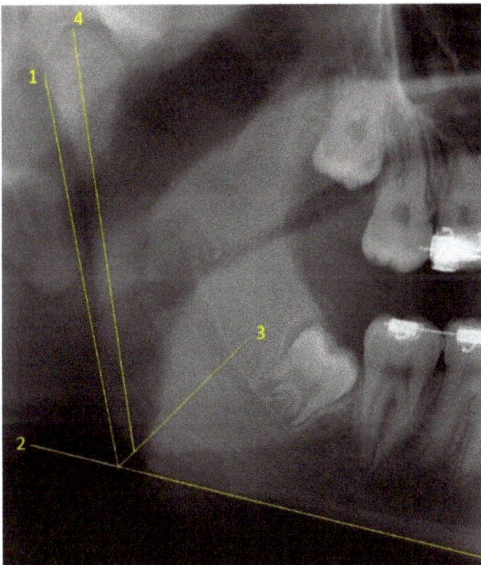

Figure 1. Ramus height measurement on the right side of the panorex using the bisection method. Lines 1 and 2 are the tangents of the mandibular ramus and the body, respectively. Line 3 is the bisection line dividing the angle between the two tangents in half. Line 4 is used to measure the ramus height and goes from the gonial angle (where line 3 crosses the curvature of the angle of the mandible, i.e., point gonion) to the highest point on the top of the condyle, i.e., point condyle.

2.2. Three-Dimensional Method

All the 3D measurements were made on segmented mandibular bones based on the CBCTs in a semi-automated way. The right side of the mandible was mirrored using Materialise ProPlan CMF 3.0 (Materialise, Leuven, Belgium), after which, it was superimposed onto the original segmentation of the left gonial angle. This area was manually selected, as shown in Figure 2. Once the observer was satisfied with the alignment, both 3D ramus shapes were exported to a standalone application created using the MATLAB R2017a (Mathworks, Natick, MA, USA) AppDesigner module. Then, the tangents of the mandibular ramus of both sides were positioned vertically, and the highest point on each condyle was marked. The difference in condylar height was equal to the vertical height difference of both points (Figure 3). All three 3D steps, i.e., segmentations, superimpositioning, and measurements, were carried out for all the patients by J.W.v.d.G., a technical physician and engineer with software experience.

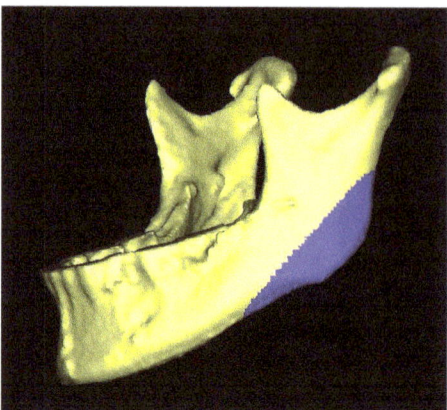

Figure 2. Three-dimensional representation of the mandibular bone. The blue surface is the area which was selected in order to align (i.e., superimpose) the original (left) and mirrored (right) mandibular angle.

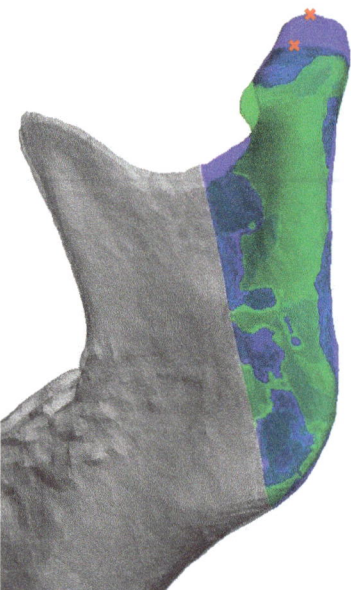

Figure 3. Three-dimensional representation of both the original (blue) as well as the aligned mirrored (green) side of the mandibular bone. The tangent of the mandibular ramus of both sides is positioned vertically, and the highest point on each condyle is marked in red. The difference in condylar height is equal to the vertical height difference of both points.

2.3. Sample Size

A pilot study with ten randomly selected patients from the orthognathic dataset was undertaken to calculate the required sample size for drawing founded conclusions when making comparisons between the 2D methods and the 3D method. The results, i.e., the mean difference between the left and right ramus height and standard deviation (data not shown), were entered in G*Power (free available Statistical Software for Power Analysis by Department of Psychology, Dusseldorf, Germany) to calculate the effect size where $p < 0.05$ and there is an acceptable power of 0.8. The required sample size for this study was determined as 32 cases. The 32 patients were randomly selected from the orthognathic dataset using the same inclusion and exclusion criteria. To test the intra- and inter-observer reliability, 10 cases were randomly selected from the group of 32. These ten cases were re-evaluated 2 weeks after the first measurements by the same observers (N.B.v.B. (2D) and J.W.v.d.G. (3D)) for intra-observer reliability. The same cases were also evaluated by different observers (F.K.L.S., an Oral and Maxillofacial surgeon specialized in TMJ surgery (2D) and J.K., a technical physician and engineer with software experience (3D)), and their measurements were compared with those made by N.B.v.B. (2D) and J.W.v.d.G. (3D) to check for inter-observer reliability. The 3D inter-observer reliability analysis involved observer J.K. performing only the last two 3D steps (see three-dimensional method above) and J.W.v.d.G. performing the segmentations.

2.4. Statistical Analysis

Statistical analyses were performed with IBM SPSS Statistics 23 (SPSS, Chicago, IL, USA). To determine if the measurements were significantly different, a paired samples *t*-test was applied. *p*-values < 0.05 were considered statistically significant. The distribution of the data was checked by constructing Q-Q plots and by performing the Kolmogorov–Smirnov test [20]. To assess the intra- and inter-observer reliability, the Intraclass Correlation Coefficients (ICC; two-way mixed effects model, single measures, absolute agreement) and the 95% confidence intervals (CI) were calculated for all 3 methods. Values less than 0.5, between 0.5 and 0.75, between 0.75 and 0.9, and larger than 0.90 were indicative of poor, moderate, good, and excellent reliability, respectively [21,22]. Bland–Altman plots were constructed to analyse measurement differences between either the observers or the repeated measurements with all three methods. The ICC results were compared; our clinically acceptable difference was 1 mm [23,24].

3. Results

The measured population (n = 32) had an average age (±s.d.) of 26.9 (±9.6) years. The cohort was made up of 59.4% (n = 19) female and 40.6% (n = 13) male patients. The average age (±s.d.) of the ten randomly selected patients for the ICC measurements was 26.5 (±7.4) years, of which 40% (n = 4) were female and 60% (n = 6) were male.

All data had a normal distribution according to the Q-Q plots and Kolmogorov–Smirnov tests (data not shown). The panorex-free-hand method showed an average difference of 2.15 mm ± 3.53 mm between the left and right ramus heights. The panorex-bisection method showed a difference of 0.93 mm ± 3.34 mm, and the CBCT measurements showed a difference of 1.41 mm ± 2.50 mm. The average absolute difference between both 2D methods was significant, 1.40 mm ± 1.10 mm ($p = 0.001$). Additionally, the panorex-bisection and CBCT measurements showed significant average differences of 1.70 mm ± 1.17 mm ($p = 0.001$). The average difference between the panorex-free-hand and the CBCT method was 1.48 mm ± 1.13 mm, which is not a significant discrepancy ($p = 0.25$).

The average differences between the first and second measurements (same observer, 2 weeks apart) was 0.85 mm ± 0.50 mm with an intra-observer reliability of 0.95 (95% CI: 0.82–0.99) for the panorex-free-hand method. Regarding the panorex-bisection, the average difference was 0.65 mm ± 0.58 mm with an intra-observer reliability of 0.95 (95% CI: 0.82–0.99). The average difference in the CBCT measurement was 0.56 mm ± 0.39 mm with an intra-observer reliability of 0.92 (95% CI: 0.73–0.98). Appendix A shows the Bland–Altman plots of all the 2D and 3D measurements.

The average measurement differences between the observers were 1.53 mm ± 0.87 mm, 0.72 mm ± 0.37 mm, and 0.76 mm ± 0.58 mm for the free-hand, the bisection, and CBCT methods, respectively (Table 1). The ICC of the inter-observer reliability of the free-hand method was 0.86 (95% CI: 0.06–0.97), the bisection method was 0.96 (95% CI: 0.78–0.99), and the CBCT method was 0.87 (95% CI: 0.56–0.97).

Table 1. Measuring results and reliability results.

	Difference in Ramus Height Left vs. Right N = 32 *	Intra-Observer Reliability N = 10 †		Inter-Observer Reliability N = 10 ‡	
Method	Mean ± SD	Mean diff ± SD	ICC (95% CI)	Mean diff ± SD	ICC (95% CI)
OPG-FH	2.15 ± 3.53	0.85 ± 0.50	0.95 (0.82–0.99)	1.53 ± 0.87	0.86 (0.06–0.97)
OPG-B	0.93 ± 3.34	0.65 ± 0.58	0.95 (0.82–0.99)	0.72 ± 0.37	0.96 (0.78–0.99)
CBCT	1.41 ± 2.50	0.56 ± 0.39	0.92 (0.73–0.98)	0.76 ± 0.58	0.87 (0.56–0.97)

* Observer N.B.v.B. performed both the OPG-FH and the OPG-B method; observer J.W.v.d.G. performed the CBCT method. † Measurements were performed 2 weeks apart by the same observers: N.B.v.B. performed both the OPG-FH and the OPG-B method; J.W.v.d.G. performed the CBCT method. ‡ Measurements performed by different observers: N.B.v.B. vs. F.K.L.S. for the OPG-FH and OPG-B method; J.W.v.d.G. vs. J.K. for the CBCT method. Abbreviations: OPG-B = two-dimensional panorex-bisection, OPG-FH = two-dimensional panorex-free-hand, CBCT = three-dimensional mirror method.

4. Discussion

Objective and reproducible measurements are key when determining the amount to resect during a proportional condylectomy in patients with active unilateral condylar hyperactivity. The aim of the study was to objectify the most reproducible ramus height measurement method when determining facial asymmetry which can be used by whomever and whenever.

A significant difference was found between the panorex-bisection and 3D measurements, as well as between the panorex-bisection and panorex-free-hand method.

The intra-observer reliability was excellent for all three methods (ICC > 0.9). The panorex-bisection also showed excellent inter-observer reliability (ICC > 0.9), while both the CBCT and panorex-free-hand gave good results (0.75 < ICC < 0.9). However, the lower boundary of the 95% CI (0.06–0.97) of the panorex-free-hand meant the inter-observer reliability was poor. Furthermore, the average difference between the inter-observer measurements of the panorex-free-hand was 1.53 mm ± 0.87 mm, which exceeds our clinically accepted margin of 1 mm. The combination of a poor lower boundary of the 95% CI of the inter-observer reliability and exceeding a clinically acceptable margin of 1 mm suggests the panorex-free-hand method is inferior for clinical use in terms of reproducible measurements of ramus height differences.

Both the 3D and bisection methods demonstrated excellent intra-observer reliability. The 3D method had a good inter-observer ICC with a moderate–excellent 95% CI, and the bisection method had an excellent inter-observer ICC with a good–excellent 95% CI. Therefore, the bisection method seems more suitable for determining mandibular ramus height differences compared to the 2D free-hand and 3D methods. Nevertheless, the most accurate display of actual asymmetry is still undetermined because there is no gold-standard, and the precise difference between the left and right ramus heights is unknown. Preferably, consecutive measurements over time, for example, in the case of a wait-and-see policy for a possibly extinguished UCH (i.e., anamnestic increasing asymmetry, but <10% difference in activity between the condyles on a SPECT image), should be performed with the bisection method because of the excellent intra-observer reliability.

Kambylafkas et al. showed that although a panorex can be used to evaluate mandibular asymmetry, some under-diagnoses will occur [17]. The panorex projection angle of the mandibular ramus in an asymmetrical mandible could differ on both sides, possibly resulting in under-diagnoses. Moreover, the position of the head of the patient while making a panorex could affect the measured asymmetry. According to Vasudeva et al. (2012), the appearance of the mandibular condyle depends on the projection angle which relates to the head's position [25]. This could negatively influence the measurements. To date, no research has reported on the influence of the projection angle on ramus height measurements. However, one could assume these factors are related and therefore the ramus height will be affected when a panorex is made at a different angle, especially in patients with UCH where the dental plane is often tilted. The patient has to bite on a piece of plastic (to position the head correctly before and during panorex-scanning), which could change the projection angle. This effect needs to be kept in mind when creating and evaluating the panorex. We hypothesize that, although our measurements were performed on a non-UCH group of patients, this will not have influenced the results of our study because reproducibility was the primary goal.

J.W.v.d.G. was the only observer who performed the CBCTs segmentations. Moerenhout et al. (2009) achieved excellent reliability on segmenting the CBCT using the Materialise software [26]. Although they used a different software, ours was also a CE-certified medical processing software (Proplan CMF), and we achieved excellent intra-observer reliability. We therefore deemed it unnecessary to repeat this step by observer J.K. to determine the inter-observer reliability.

Markic et al. (2015) were also able to make reliable ramus height measurements on panorex and CBCT images [9] and found excellent intra- and inter-observer reliabilities for both imaging modalities, indicating they can be used to measure asymmetry. Their measuring method was slightly different to ours as both Co and Go were constructed in a different way: Co was the intersection point of the tangent with the condyle of a line perpendicular to the tangent of the posterior border of the mandible. Hence, the Co was not the most cranial point of the condyle, but lower and more posterior. We are not sure if it is possible to correct for this when performing a proportional condylectomy, i.e., resectioning the most cranial part of the condyle. We consider this to be a tricky situation, especially when the condyle is greatly inclined anteriorly. Markic et al.'s Go point was the intersection point of the lower border of the line through Co parallel to the tangent of the posterior border of the mandible. We hypothesize that with an increasing high mandibular plane angle, and/or as the inclination of the condyle increases, the Go point will be located more anteriorly. Furthermore, their sample size was smaller, no power analyses were performed, and a 95% CI was not reported. Our Go point was the same as that described by Gaufield: a point on the curvature of the angle of the mandible located by bisecting the angle formed by lines tangent to the posterior ramus and the inferior border of the mandible [16].

Nolte et al. performed a 3D quantification of mandibular asymmetry in 37 UCH patients and compared this with a group of healthy subjects, matched for age and gender. It is unclear why they had this number of subjects. They concluded that CBCT is a useful and accurate modality for this purpose [19]. Although they performed linear measurements on the data, they did not make any comparisons with 2D methods. In another study of patients with unilateral condylar hyperplasia, Nolte et al. performed measurements on panoramic radiographs [27]. They subdivided their measurements into condylar head, condylar neck, ramus height, angle of gonion, and body height. They defined the ramus height as "the total length between the most upper and lower points perpendicular to the tangential line of the mandibular ramus". It is not completely clear to us how this was carried out. Nevertheless, the biggest difference in between-observer reproducibility was observed for the condylar head and condylar neck measurements. Regarding the ramus height, they found a difference between the affected and healthy side: the between-observer reproducibility (kappa), as assessed on an orthopantomogram, was 0.88 for the affected side and 0.96 for the healthy side. A power analysis was not performed by that study, and therefore, firm conclusions cannot be drawn.

Sembronio et al. also performed 3D virtual mirroring by superimposing the contralateral healthy side on the condylar hyperplasia side [28]. A custom-designed condylar cutting guide was modelled on the condylar head, allowing for the precise tracing of the osteotomy as planned. This technique proved to be very useful for the seven patients treated in this way. However, the paper did not give any information about the accuracy of the planned and performed condylectomy. Combining the most reproducible and the most accurate measuring method with the guided surgery, as described by Sembronio et al., is potentially a suitable method for correcting asymmetry and should be part of future studies.

A substantial difference of 1.70 mm ± 1.17 mm was found by us between the panorex-bisection and 3D measurements, which means there was a clinically relevant (>1 mm) discrepancy between them. All the patients with more than a two-millimetre difference between measurements (which was the case with 10 of the 32 cases in total) were closely reviewed. No explanation could be found for three of the ten cases. In the other seven cases, it was difficult to identify the mandibular angle, the highest point of the condyle, or both, on the panorex image because of overprojection with other structures. Nevertheless, the intra- and inter-observer reliabilities of the panorex-bisection method were both higher compared to the 3D measurements. This indicates that the repeatability of the measurements is better, but that the accuracy of the measurements compared to the actual asymmetry is questionable in the presence of overprojection, making it difficult to identify the mandibular angle and/or the top of the condyle.

To the best of our knowledge, comparisons of different measuring methods for ramus height involving power analyses, as was performed in our study, has never been described in the available literature. This research provides a better understanding of (1) the reliability of the currently available and easily accessible 2D methods, resulting in us switching from the panorex-free-hand to the panorex-bisection method in daily practice, and (2) the possible contribution of 3D to proportional condylectomy surgery, which is promising considering the 3D method is still in an early phase of development. The most accurate display of the actual asymmetry remains undetermined because there is no gold-standard and because the precise difference between left and right ramus heights is unknown. More research needs to be carried out to determine this, including developing an easy, quick-to-use, and more reliable method for daily practice based on (CB)CTs, e.g., the use of fully automatic (1) mandible segmentations, (2) superimposition algorithms, and (3) ramus height difference measurements.

In conclusion, we discourage the use of the panorex-free-hand method in clinical use for reproducibility measurements of ramus height differences. The two-dimensional panorex-bisection method is the most reliable method, provided that the panorex images are good quality.

Author Contributions: Conceptualization, N.B.v.B., J.K. and F.K.L.S.; methodology, N.B.v.B., J.W.v.d.G. and J.K.; validation, J.W.v.d.G. and J.K.; formal Analysis, N.B.v.B., J.W.v.d.G., J.K. and F.K.L.S.; investigation, J.W.v.d.G.; writing—original draft preparation, N.B.v.B. and J.W.v.d.G.; writing—review and editing, N.B.v.B., J.W.v.d.G., J.K. and F.K.L.S.; Supervision, J.K. All authors have read and agreed to the published version of the manuscript.

Funding: This research received no external funding.

Institutional Review Board Statement: The study was conducted in accordance with the Declaration of Helsinki, and approved by the Institutional Review Board (or Ethics Committee) of the University Medical Center Groningen, the Netherlands.

Informed Consent Statement: Not applicable.

Data Availability Statement: The data described in this study are available in Table 1, Figures 1–3 and Appendix A. The raw data presented in this study are available on request from the corresponding author. Requests for materials should be addressed to N.B.v.B.

Conflicts of Interest: The authors declare no conflict of interest.

Appendix A. Bland–Altman Plots of All the Intra- and Inter-Observer Tests

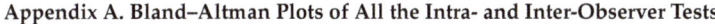

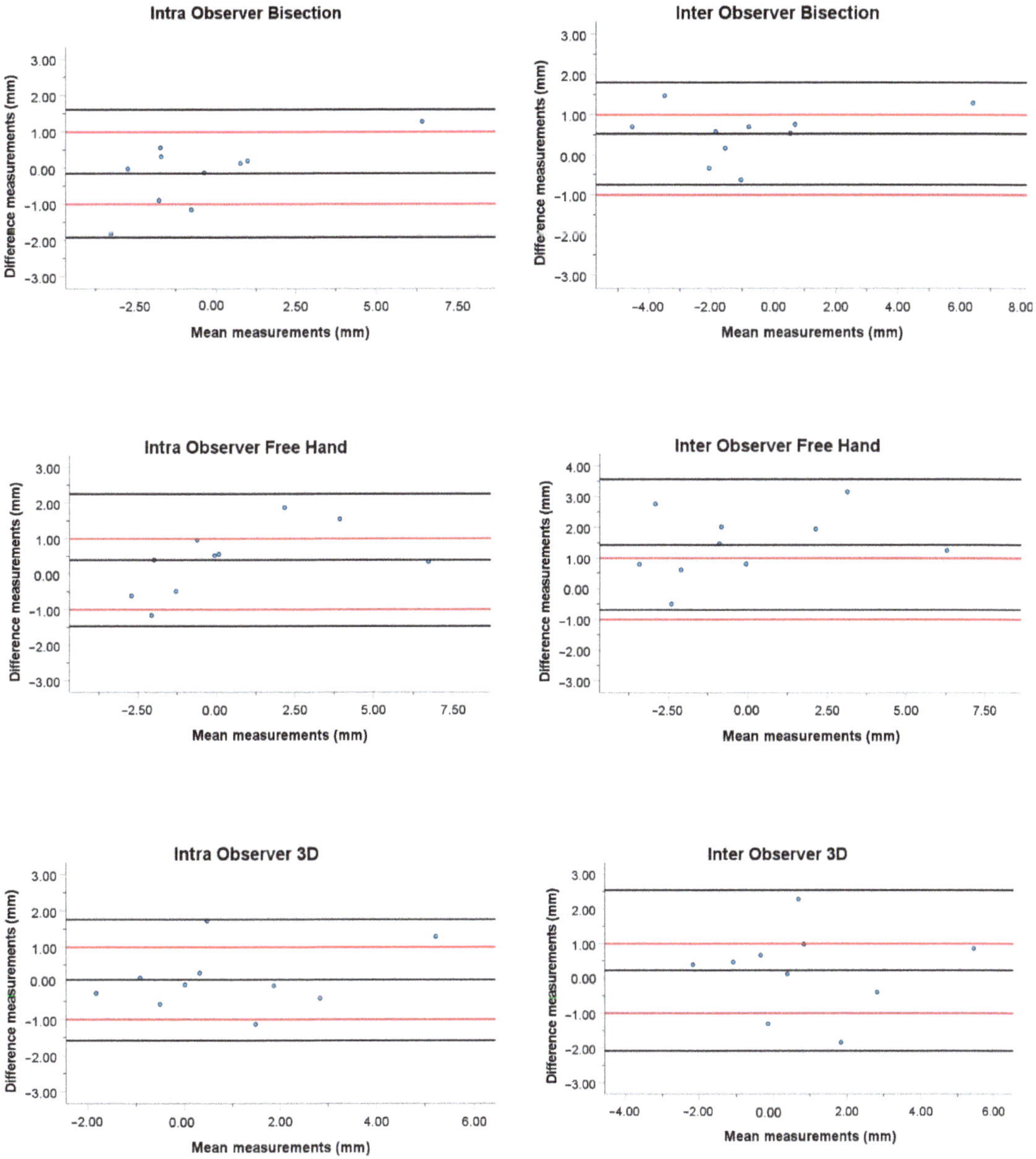

Figure A1. The *x*-axis in all the plots represents the mean of both measurements (mm) but does not say anything about the accuracy because there is no gold-standard, and the actual difference between left and right ramus heights is unknown. The *y*-axis show the difference between both measurements (intra-observer) and both observers (inter-observer) (mm). The black lines represent the 95% confidence intervals (upper and lower black lines) and the average of the measurements (middle black line). The red lines represent our clinically acceptable measurement error of 1 mm.

References

1. Obwegeser, H.L.; Makek, M.S. Hemimandibular hyperplasia–hemimandibular elongation. *J. Maxillofac. Surg.* **1986**, *14*, 183–208. [CrossRef]
2. Karssemakers, L.H.E. Unilaterale condylaire hyperactiviteit. *Ned. Tijdschr. Tandheelkd.* **2012**, *119*, 500–504. [CrossRef] [PubMed]
3. Saridin, C.P.; Raijmakers, P.G.H.M.; Tuinzing, D.B.; Becking, A.G. Comparison of planar bone scintigraphy and single photon emission computed tomography in patients suspected of having unilateral condylar hyperactivity. *Oral Surg. Oral Med. Oral Pathol. Oral Radiol. Endodontol.* **2008**, *106*, 426–432. [CrossRef] [PubMed]
4. Maniskas, S.A.; Ly, C.L.; Pourtaheri, N.; Parsaei, Y.; Steinbacher, D.M. Concurrent High Condylectomy and Orthognathic Surgery for Treatment of Patients with Unilateral Condylar Hyperplasia. *J. Craniofac. Surg.* **2020**, *31*, 2217–2221. [CrossRef]
5. Almeida, L.E.; Zacharias, J.; Pierce, S. Condylar hyperplasia: An updated review of the literature. *Korean J. Orthod.* **2015**, *45*, 333–340. [CrossRef]
6. Mouallem, G.; Vernex-Boukerma, Z.; Longis, J.; Perrin, J.P.; Delaire, J.; Mercier, J.M.; Corre, P. Efficacy of proportional condylectomy in a treatment protocol for unilateral condylar hyperplasia: A review of 73 cases. *J. Cranio-Maxillofac. Surg.* **2017**, *45*, 1083–1093. [CrossRef]
7. Fariña, R.; Olate, S.; Raposo, A.; Araya, I.; Alister, J.P.; Uribe, F. High condylectomy versus proportional condylectomy: Is secondary orthognathic surgery necessary? *Int. J. Oral Maxillofac. Surg.* **2016**, *45*, 72–77. [CrossRef]
8. Niño-Sandoval, T.C.; Maia, F.P.A.; Vasconcelos, B.C.E. Efficacy of proportional versus high condylectomy in active condylar hyperplasia—A systematic review. *J. Cranio-Maxillofac. Surg.* **2019**, *47*, 1222–1232. [CrossRef]
9. Markic, G.; Müller, L.; Patcas, R.; Roos, M.; Lochbühler, N.; Peltomäki, T.; Karlo, C.A.; Ullrich, O.; Kellenberger, C.J. Assessing the length of the mandibular ramus and the condylar process: A comparison of OPG, CBCT, CT, MRI, and lateral cephalometric measurements. *Eur. J. Orthod.* **2015**, *37*, 13–21. [CrossRef]
10. Türp, J.C.; Vach, W.; Harbich, K.; Alt, K.W.; Strub, J.R. Determining mandibular condyle and ramus height with the help of an Orthopantomogram®—A valid method? *J. Oral Rehabil.* **1996**, *23*, 395–400. [CrossRef]
11. de Oliveira, F.T.; Soares, M.Q.S.; Sarmento, V.A.; Rubira, C.M.F.; Lauris, J.R.P.; Rubira-Bullen, I.R.F. Mandibular ramus length as an indicator of chronological age and sex. *Int. J. Legal Med.* **2014**, *129*, 195–201. [CrossRef] [PubMed]
12. Laster, W.S.; Ludlow, J.B.; Bailey, L.J.; Hershey, H.G. Accuracy of measurements of mandibular anatomy and prediction of asymmetry in panoramic radiographic images. *Dentomaxillofacial Radiol.* **2005**, *34*, 343–349. [CrossRef] [PubMed]
13. Kjellberg, H.; Ekestubbe, A.; Kiliaridis, S.; Thilander, B. Condylar height on panoramic radiographs: A methodologic study with a clinical application. *Acta Odontol. Scand.* **1994**, *52*, 43–50. [CrossRef] [PubMed]
14. Puricelli, E. Panorametry: Suggestion of a method for mandibular measurements on panoramic radiographs. *Head Face Med.* **2009**, *5*, 19. [CrossRef]
15. Parma, C. Die Röntgendiagnostik der Kiefergelenke. *Röntgenpraxis* **1932**, *7*, 633–639.
16. Caufield, P.W. Tracing Technique and Identification of Landmarks. In *Radiographic Cephalometry, from Basics to 3-D Imaging*; Jacobson, A., Jacobson, R.L., Eds.; Quintessence Books; Quintessence Pub. Co.: Berlin, Germany, 2006.
17. Kambylafkas, P.; Murdock, E.; Gilda, E.; Tallents, R.H.; Kyrkanides, S. Validity of panoramic radiographs for measuring mandibular asymmetry. *Angle Orthod.* **2006**, *76*, 388–393. [CrossRef]
18. De Bont, L.G.M.; van der Kuijl, B.; Stegenga, B.; Vencken, L.M.; Boering, G. Computed tomography in differential diagnosis of temporomandibular joint disorders. *Int. J. Oral Maxillofac. Surg.* **1993**, *22*, 200–209. [CrossRef]
19. Nolte, J.W.; Verhoeven, T.J.; Schreurs, R.; Bergé, S.J.; Karssemakers, L.H.E.; Becking, A.G.; Maal, T.J.J. 3-Dimensional CBCT analysis of mandibular asymmetry in unilateral condylar hyperplasia. *J. Cranio-Maxillofac. Surg.* **2016**, *44*, 1970–1976. [CrossRef]
20. Field, A. *Discovering Statistics Using IBM SPSS Statistics*; SAGE Publications Ltd.: Thousand Oaks, CA, USA, 2005.
21. Koo, T.K.; Li, M.Y. A Guideline of Selecting and Reporting Intraclass Correlation Coefficients for Reliability Research. *J. Chiropr. Med.* **2016**, *15*, 155–163. [CrossRef]
22. Nunnally, J.C.; Bernstein, I.H. *Psychometric Theory*; McGraw-Hill Series in Psychology: New York, NY, USA, 1994; p. 583.
23. Van den Bempt, M.; Liebregts, J.; Maal, T.; Bergé, S.; Xi, T. Toward a higher accuracy in orthognathic surgery by using intraoperative computer navigation, 3D surgical guides, and/or customized osteosynthesis plates: A systematic review. *J. Cranio-Maxillofac. Surg.* **2018**, *46*, 2108–2119. [CrossRef]
24. Almukhtar, A.; Ju, X.; Khambay, B.; McDonald, J.; Ayoub, A. Comparison of the accuracy of voxel based registration and surface based registration for 3D assessment of surgical change following orthognathic surgery. *PLoS ONE* **2014**, *9*, e93402. [CrossRef] [PubMed]
25. Beloor Vasudeva, S.; Kameko, N.; Endo, A.; Okano, T. Influence of horizontal condylar angle and X-ray projection angle on the appearance of the condyle on lateral temporomandibular joint panoramic radiographs. *Oral Health Dent. Manag.* **2012**, *11*, 177–184. [PubMed]
26. Moerenhout, B.A.M.M.L.; Gelaude, F.; Swennen, G.; Casselman, J.; Van Der Sloten, J.; Mommaerts, M. Accuracy and repeatability of cone-beam computed tomography (CBCT) measurements used in the determination of facial indices in the laboratory setup. *J. Craniomaxillofac. Surg.* **2008**, *37*, 18–23. [CrossRef] [PubMed]

27. Nolte, J.W.; Karssemakers, L.H.E.; Grootendorst, D.C.; Tuinzing, D.B.; Becking, A.G. Panoramic imaging is not suitable for quantitative evaluation, classification, and follow up in unilateral condylar hyperplasia. *Br. J. Oral Maxillofac. Surg.* **2015**, *53*, 446–450. [CrossRef] [PubMed]
28. Sembronio, S.; Tel, A.; Costa, F.; Robiony, M. An Updated Protocol for the Treatment of Condylar Hyperplasia: Computer-Guided Proportional Condylectomy. *J. Oral Maxillofac. Surg.* **2019**, *77*, 1457–1465. [CrossRef]

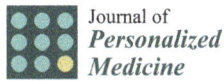

Article

The Accuracy of Patient-Specific Spinal Drill Guides Is Non-Inferior to Computer-Assisted Surgery: The Results of a Split-Spine Randomized Controlled Trial

Peter A. J. Pijpker [1,2,*], Jos M. A. Kuijlen [1], Katalin Tamási [1,3], D. L. Marinus Oterdoom [1], Rob A. Vergeer [1], Gijs Rijtema [1], Maarten H. Coppes [1], Joep Kraeima [2,4] and Rob J. M. Groen [1]

1. Department of Neurosurgery, University Medical Center Groningen, University of Groningen, 9700 RB Groningen, The Netherlands; j.m.a.kuijlen@umcg.nl (J.M.A.K.); k.tamasi@umcg.nl (K.T.); d.l.m.oterdoom@umcg.nl (D.L.M.O.); ra.vergeer@umcg.nl (R.A.V.); g.rijtema@umcg.nl (G.R.); m.h.coppes@umcg.nl (M.H.C.); r.j.m.groen@umcg.nl (R.J.M.G.)
2. 3D-Lab, University Medical Center Groningen, University of Groningen, 9700 RB Groningen, The Netherlands; j.kraeima@umcg.nl
3. Department of Epidemiology, University Medical Center Groningen, 9700 RB Groningen, The Netherlands
4. Department of Oral and Maxillofacial Surgery, University Medical Center Groningen, University of Groningen, 9700 RB Groningen, The Netherlands
* Correspondence: p.a.j.pijpker@umcg.nl

Abstract: In recent years, patient-specific spinal drill guides (3DPGs) have gained widespread popularity. Several studies have shown that the accuracy of screw insertion with these guides is superior to that obtained using the freehand insertion technique, but there are no studies that make a comparison with computer-assisted surgery (CAS). The aim of this study was to determine whether the accuracy of insertion of spinal screws using 3DPGs is non-inferior to insertion via CAS. A randomized controlled split-spine study was performed in which 3DPG and CAS were randomly assigned to the left or right sides of the spines of patients undergoing fixation surgery. The 3D measured accuracy of screw insertion was the primary study outcome parameter. Sixty screws inserted in 10 patients who completed the study protocol were used for the non-inferiority analysis. The non-inferiority of 3DPG was demonstrated for entry-point accuracy, as the upper margin of the 95% CI (−1.01 mm–0.49 mm) for the difference between the means did not cross the predetermined non-inferiority margin of 1 mm ($p < 0.05$). We also demonstrated non-inferiority of 3D angular accuracy ($p < 0.05$), with a 95% CI for the true difference of $-2.30°$–$1.35°$, not crossing the predetermined non-inferiority margin of 3° ($p < 0.05$). The results of this randomized controlled trial (RCT) showed that 3DPGs provide a non-inferior alternative to CAS in terms of screw insertion accuracy and have considerable potential as a navigational technique in spinal fixation.

Keywords: spine surgery; virtual surgical planning (VSP); 3D-printing; patient-specific instrumentation; drill guides; computer-assisted surgery; image-guided surgery; image-guided navigation; pedicle screw; lateral mass screw

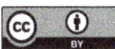

1. Introduction

Spinal instability is commonly treated through surgical fixation involving vertebral screw insertion. Conditions that frequently result in spinal instability are fractures after trauma, spinal deformities, tumors, and degenerative diseases. Spinal fixation is aimed at gaining stability and preventing subsequent neurological deficit. Generally, the bilateral positioning of screws in the vertebrae around the level(s) of instability is needed to achieve the immobilization of the unstable segments. The accurate insertion of screws is essential for achieving safe and optimal spinal fixation surgery. Conversely, malpositioned screws can induce damage of vital structures or result in the failure of fixation [1,2].

Traditionally, freehand insertion of screws is performed according to anatomical landmarks and through fluoroscopy control. However, because freehand screw insertion does not account for structural variations, including anatomical variance or severe deformations, there is an increased risk of malpositioned screws and related neurovascular complications [3–6]. Advances in spinal surgery have led to the development of computer-assisted surgery (CAS) navigation systems, also often mentioned as image-guided surgery, or intraoperative navigation. Initially, CAS systems relied on preoperative CT, which had to be manually re-registered for each individual vertebra and was associated with substantial registration errors. With the advent of modern CAS systems that rely on intraoperative acquired CT, this time-consuming repetitive calibration for individual vertebrae became redundant, leading to the increased use of CAS in spinal surgery. The accuracy of screw insertion has been substantially improved with current CAS systems, with a significantly reduced misplacement rate compared with the misplacement rate associated with freehand screw insertion [7,8]. Although spine surgeons with specific subspecialties (e.g., minimally invasive surgery and oncology) have widely incorporated CAS into their practices, the technology has not been adopted in all hospitals. In addition, the accuracy of screw insertion in cases with a highly mobile cervical spine reportedly fails to meet the high accuracy that is achieved in other spinal areas, which is most likely induced by the intraoperative shifting of segments. Moreover, despite these modern techniques, screw malpositioning does still occur, with the reported prevalence of malpositions being as high as 19% [9,10]. For these reasons, there is an ongoing demand for alternative navigational technologies that can be used to facilitate accurate spinal screw insertion.

Recent developments in medical computer-aided design and manufacturing techniques have given rise to completely new methods of surgical planning, commonly referred to as 3D virtual surgical planning (VSP) and patient-specific instrumentation (PSI) technology. The PSI technology comprises 3D-printed instrumentation that allows for the translation of the VSP to surgery. PSI are currently widely applied within different specialties [11], and the use of 3D-printed drill guides (3DPGs) has been attracting increasing attention as a promising navigational tool for spinal screw insertion. Recent studies have shown that 3DPGs are feasible for cervical and thoracic spine instrumentation, as demonstrated in cadaveric studies [12–17] and in clinical trials [18–23]. Moreover, their specific applications have been described for scoliosis surgery [24,25], C2 lamina screw insertion [26], and C1–C2 transarticular screw insertion [27]. Compared with CAS, the 3DPGs have several advantages. First, it provides the benefit of having a preformulated screw plan that includes the direction, length, and thickness of the screws. Second, it eliminates the need for intraoperative fluoroscopy. Third, it is applied to individual vertebra and is thus unaffected by intervertebral motion, which, in the case of CAS, can lead to workflow interruptions resulting from re-registration. Fourth, 3DPGs do not induce a surgical line of sight interference as in the case with CAS, which requires to constant looking back and forth between the patient and the screen. Last, 3DPGs do not require costly hospital investments.

The findings of various studies reported in the literature that have directly compared the accuracy of freehand and 3DPG screw insertion have all demonstrated the superiority of guides over the freehand technique [28–30]. However, comparisons of CAS and 3DPG are sparse within the literature; only one study has compared groups of patients instrumented with 3DPG and CAS [31]. To the best of our knowledge, a randomized comparative study of 3DPG and CAS has not been previously conducted.

Although 3DPGs appear to have several advantages, to become accepted as a viable alternative navigational tool its accuracy must first be shown to be comparable to that of CAS. Consequently, the objective of this randomized trial was to demonstrate the non-inferiority of 3DPG relative to CAS in terms of the accuracy of pedicle and lateral mass screw insertion.

2. Materials and Methods

2.1. Study Design

The SpineGuides study was a single-center, prospective, investigator-driven study that randomly allocated screws to either 3DPG or CAS-assisted instrumentation in patients undergoing clinically indicated fixation surgery. All consecutive patients scheduled for cervical and/or thoracic spinal fixation surgery were eligible for this study. Exclusion criteria were: (1) patients aged below 16 years, (2) scoliosis surgery, (3) previous surgical history entailing laminectomy or the application of osteosynthesis material at the target levels, (4) urgent cases, and (5) unilateral instrumentation. This trial was undertaken after obtaining approval from the ethical board of the local medical institution (ref no. M19.229543). Written informed consent was obtained from each patient prior to their enrollment in the study. The trial has been registered on euclinicaltrials.eu with a registration number of 2022-500880-11-00.

The study was designed to determine whether the accuracy of screw insertion in spinal fixation surgery performed with the 3DPG navigational technique is non-inferior relative to that of screw insertion performed using the CAS technique. Because spinal bone geometry, density, and microstructure can vary widely among subjects, a "split-spine" design was selected for the study. The two navigational techniques were randomly assigned to either the left or the right side of the spinal column. The split-spine design removed the influence of interindividual variability in the study arms and also ensured that vertebral levels and screw insertion techniques (mass lateral vs. pedicle) were evenly distributed.

The two techniques were randomly assigned to the right or left side of the spinal column by generating balanced permutations via computer randomization. The randomization was constrained by blocks such that an equal number of techniques per side are obtained. The inclusion was limited to bilateral screw insertion, which resulted in a consistent number of screws at each vertebral level within both study groups. The randomization scheme was created using the online tool at randomization.com (http://www.randomization.com, accessed on 5 January 2019) prior to commencing the study, and randomization codes were enclosed in sealed envelopes.

2.2. Virtual Surgical Planning

Virtual surgical planning (VSP) was carried out in accordance with a previously developed workflow, and 3DPGs were fabricated according to our previously published blueprint [17,23]. The brief description of the VSP and PSI steps are as follows. First, the preoperative CT was imported into medical image data segmentation software (Mimics, Materialise, Leuven, Belgium). Threshold-based segmentation was performed for each vertebral level to obtain 3D anatomical models, and optimal trajectories were manually defined. Then, 3DPGs were designed and manufactured in polyamide in accordance with ISO 13,485 standards and sterilized for intraoperative use by autoclave steam sterilization. Knowledge of the allocation was concealed from the 3D-specialist (PP) in charge of planning screw trajectories and designing the guides.

2.3. Surgical Technique

The standard surgical procedure was applied, starting cranially and continuing caudally placing screws sequentially at each level. Because randomization was concealed from the 3D specialist, the 3DPGs were designed with bilateral drill holes. Therefore, they would only fit if screws had not yet been inserted at the level of interest. Accordingly, for each level to be instrumented, the protocol stated to start with the 3DPG-assigned side followed by the contralateral CAS-assigned side. The 3DPGs were positioned after performing meticulous removal of soft tissue. Pilot holes (2 mm) were drilled at high-speed using appropriate drill stops (Figure 1). In the case of thick screws, the trajectories were enlarged/expanded using a straight pedicle probe. The study protocol ensured that the 3DPG burr hole checking was not performed using the CAS system, in order to keep the study arms separate. For the CAS study arm, the screw trajectories were created according to the standard CAS guiding procedure applied at our neurosurgical department, which consists of several steps. The steps applied in the CAS-assisted screw placement were as follows: (1) entry point identification using the CAS pointer and its marking with a ball-tipped burr, (2) definition of an optimal trajectory using the pointer, and (3) creation of a burr hole through alternated probing (or drilling for lateral mass) and pointer-based checking until the desired trajectory was achieved. For the purposes of this study, the ultimate CAS trajectory was saved intraoperatively by positioning the CAS pointer in the drill hole and storing the trajectory's coordinates within the system. By opening the saved data using the CAS cranial module (instead of the regular spine module) postoperatively, we were able to retrieve the trajectory's coordinates in the digital imaging and communications in medicine (DICOM) format (Figure 2). The cone-shaped pointer tip ensured concentric positioning within the drill hole. During the procedure, no navigated drill or screwdriver was used, as these tools were not part of our center's standard procedure, nor it was available within the collection of instruments. The CAS setting comprised a mobile Arcadis Orbic 3D fluoroscopy C-arm (Siemens Medical Solutions, Erlangen, Germany) combined with a Brainlab optical navigation system (BrainLab Curve, BrainLAB, Munich, Germany).

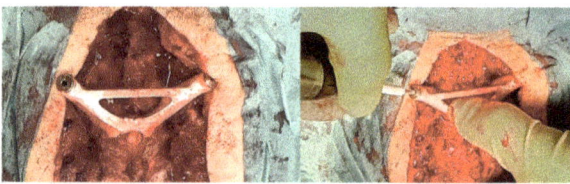

Figure 1. 3DPG positioning and high-speed pilot hole drilling. A drill stop was slid over the drill bit to prevent penetration of the anterior cortex.

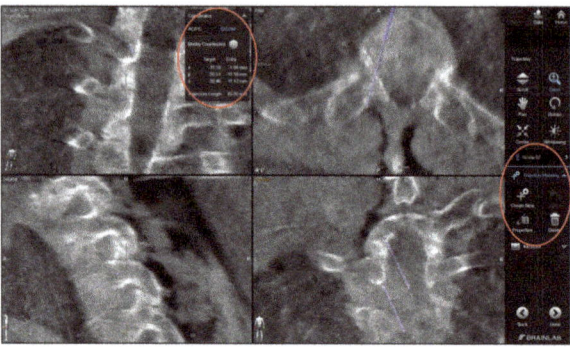

Figure 2. Retrieval of the DICOM coordinates of the intraoperatively stored trajectories accomplished by opening the spine planning file inside the cranial module of the planning software.

2.4. Outcome Measures

The accuracy of the primary radiological screw insertion was the main parameter assessed in this study. Accuracy was measured by the amount of deviation from the plan using two continuous variables: (1) deviation from planned entry point (in mm); and (2) the 3D angular deviation (in degrees) from the planned trajectory. For the 3DPG arm, the deviation was measured following level-by-level registration of the postoperative CT with the preoperative CT, which included the planned trajectories. For the CAS study arm, the postoperative CT was registered with the intraoperative CT, which included the stored CAS trajectories (Figure 3). As a result of the registration per vertebra (single-level registration of each vertebra), the patient's alignment (supine vs. prone) and spinal mobility did not affect the final analysis.

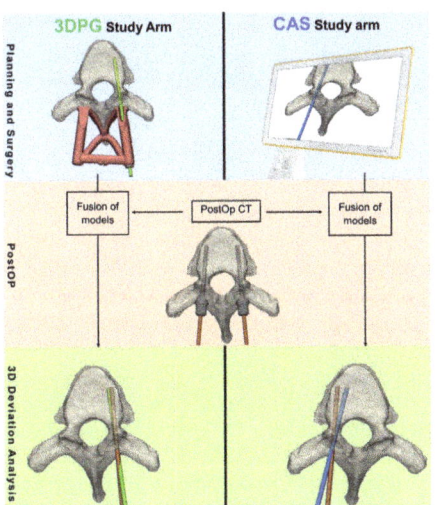

Figure 3. Schematic overview of the study depicting preoperative planning, preoperative measurements, and postoperative assessment procedures. 3DPG: 3D printed guides; CAS: Computer assisted surgery; 3D: 3 dimensional; PostOp CT: postoperative CT.

During the analysis, computerized registration and measurements were performed wherever possible. In technical terms, this procedure entailed (1) automated surface-based model registration using the Iterative Closest Point algorithm and (2) the use of automatically fitted analytical cylinders at the screw positions. These cylinders were automatically placed over the screw objects to prevent any assessment bias. Screw segmentation was done using standardized Hounsfield thresholds to eliminate bias by segmentation. The 3D deviation analysis has previously been shown to have very high inter-rater reliability, with an intraclass correlation coefficient of 0.99 [23].

2.5. Statistics

The objective of this study was to assess the non-inferiority of the 3DPG navigational technique relative to CAS. The calculation of the sample size was based on preselected margins of non-inferiority: 1 mm for entry-point accuracy and 3° for angular accuracy. In order to obtain representative margins and in the absence of representative published 3D deviation data, we conducted a small, pilot 3D simulation in which we measured the maximum amount of screw rotation until pedicle wall breach occurred. The upper limit of the rotation in which 99% of screws fitted within the pedicle was calculated as 3.29°. The allowable margins of error for screw placement reported in the literature are around 1 mm and 5°, respectively, for translation and rotation [32,33]. Although the metrics reported in the literature and those obtained in our pilot experiment were slightly different, they were in line with our predetermined margins. Hence, we concluded that they justified our selected margins of non-inferiority.

The sample size of each group was calculated according to the accuracy data derived from our pilot study along with additional pilot data gathered during CAS-assisted surgery. Because the current study focused solely on radiological accuracy outcomes obtained through 3D deviation analysis and because we assumed that the screws were independent, we calculated the screw-based sample size. Applying our assumptions in the calculation of sample size, we found that 36 screws demonstrated 90% power for determining non-inferiority at a significance level of 0.05. To compensate for unanticipated problems such as loss to follow up and equipment malformation, we included a dropout of 10% and therefore aimed to include a minimum of 40 screws (20 in each study arm). Considering the average number of cervical screws used per patient in our center, we aimed to include

10 patients in the study. The power calculation was performed using PASS software (NCSS, LLC, Kaysville, UT, USA).

All of the accuracy data were presented as descriptive statistics, expressed as median and interquartile range IQR values for non-normal distributed parameters. Non-inferiority was assessed by calculating the mean and 95% CI values for the difference between the 3DPG and CAS using a one-sample t-test and comparing the limits of the CI with predefined non-inferiority margins. The decision to reject the null hypothesis was made by determining whether the upper bound of the CI crossed the non-inferiority margin.

The final statistical analysis was performed using the SPSS Statistics program (SPSS Version 23.0 for Windows, IBM, N, Armonk, NY, USA).

3. Results

3.1. Patient Characteristics

Between June 2019 and December 2020, all of the consecutive patients referred for multi-level cervical and thoracic spine fixation were prospectively enrolled. A total of 10 patients were initially enrolled to meet the sample size calculations. A loss of CAS trajectory data due to storage failure, which exceeded the calculated dropout rate, resulted in the enrolment of three additional patients after approval by the institutional board had been renewed. Altogether, the number of patients suitable for the final analysis was 10. Because the ultimate number of screws inserted per patients turned out to be higher than expected, the final number of screws per study arm was 30.

The mean age of all patients was 56 years (range 16–82) and 5 of the 10 patients were women. The cohort presented with a spectrum of indications, including degenerative disease, osteoporotic fractures, rheumatoid arthritis, Klippel–Feil syndrome, and tumor.

3.2. Descriptive Statistics

The median entry point deviation was 1.8 mm (IQR: 1.0 mm–2.9 mm) in the cohort instrumented with 3DPG, and 1.8 mm (IQR: 1.0 mm–3.2 mm) in the cohort instrumented with CAS. The angular deviation was 5.7° (IQR: 2.9°–9.1°) in the cohort instrumented with 3DPG and 5.3° (IQR: 3.8°–8.1°) in the cohort instrumented with CAS (Figure 4).

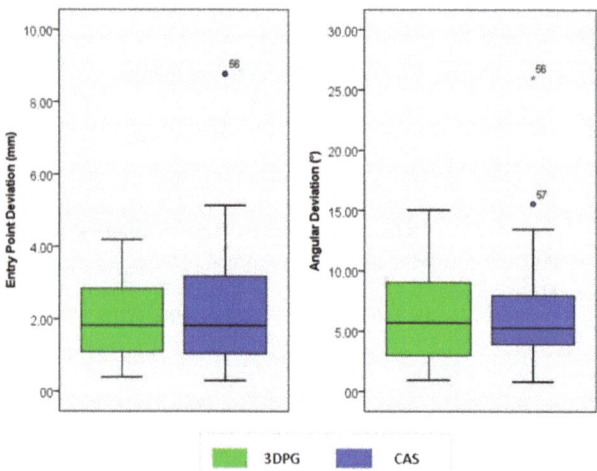

Figure 4. Entry point deviation (in mm) and angular deviation (in °) for screws used in the 3DPG (green) and CAS (blue) study groups.

3.3. Non-Inferiority Assessment

The 95% confidence interval (CI) for the difference in means between 3DPG and CAS (3DPG-CAS) was −1.01 mm to 0.49 mm. Therefore, the entry-point accuracy of 3DPG demonstrated non-inferiority relative to CAS, as the upper margin of the CI did not cross the predetermined non-inferiority margin of 1 mm ($p < 0.05$), which has been visualized in Figure 5. For angular accuracy, the 95% CI for the true difference between the means was −2.30° to 1.35°. Therefore, the angular accuracy of 3DPG was also found to be non-inferior relative to CAS, as the upper margin of the CI did not cross the predetermined non-inferiority margin of 3° ($p < 0.05$) (Figure 5).

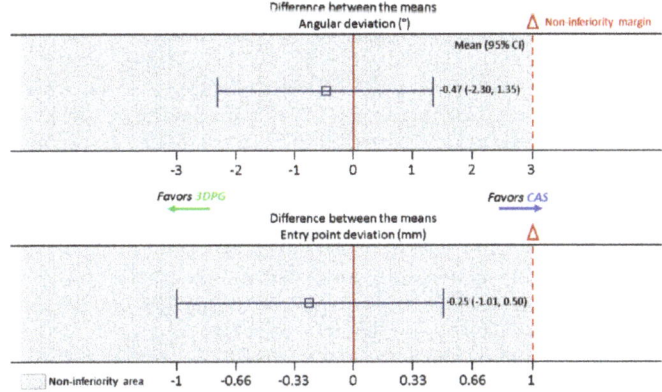

Figure 5. Graph displaying non-inferiority of 3DPG (test) relative to CAS (active control). The error bars demonstrate two-sided CIs, displaying both the lower and upper bounds of the CI. For both outcome measures, 3DPG was non-inferior relative to CAS, given that the entire CI was below the predetermined non-inferiority margins (Δ). It should be noted that a smaller outcome value (less deviation) indicated a better outcome. Therefore, areas to the left indicated better outcomes, and areas to the right indicated worse outcomes.

4. Discussion

In this prospective randomized clinical trial (RCT), we compared the accuracy of spinal screw insertion using 3DPG and CAS. Our results showed that screw insertion accuracy achieved using 3DPG was similar and non-inferior to that obtained with CAS.

To the best of our knowledge, this RCT is the first to compare the accuracy of spinal screw insertion using 3DPG and CAS. Previous studies have compared 3DPG and freehand screw insertion, with their findings leading to a general consensus that the 3DPG technology significantly reduces the incidence of pedicle screw malpositioning [29,30]. Moreover, significant reductions in radiation exposure and in the time taken for screw implantation using this technology have been reported [28]. We only found one study by Fan et al. that compared groups of patients instrumented with CAS and 3DPG [31]. This prospective cohort study compared the use of robot-assisted pedicle screw insertion with 3DPG, CAS, and free-hand fluoroscopy-controlled screw insertion. The study demonstrated that the accuracy of "acceptable" screw placement in the 3DPG-guided group (95.52%) was slightly higher than that in the CAS group (90.60%), with no significant difference found between the two groups. These results suggest that both techniques yield similar degrees of accuracy; however, a systematic, randomized comparison was not performed in the above study. It is generally acknowledged that pedicle screw insertion has been substantially improved through the use of CAS technology compared with free-hand screw insertion. Hence, it was our belief that this accuracy standard should be the reference for novel navigational technologies such as 3DPG. Therefore, to become accepted as viable navigational tool and to optimize safety, an RCT should be conducted between 3DPG and CAS with the aim of determining, at minimum, non-inferior screw insertion accuracy, as was done in the current study.

The results of our randomized study indicated similar degrees of accuracy for both techniques. Compared with the accuracy of CAS, that of 3DPG was non-inferior for both of the assessed parameters. In fact, the upper limits of our 95% CI were 0.50 mm and 1.35°, which were well below the respective non-inferiority limits of 1 mm and 3°. There was no indication of 3DPG being superior to CAS, as the CI upper limits were above zero. However, we believe that a sufficiently powered study could lead to a finding of the superiority of 3DPG in specific subgroups. In particular, the use of CAS in the highly mobile upper cervical spine may be associated with increasing errors when operating further away from the reference array, with surgical manipulation inducing slight realignments of vertebral levels [34]. As our study design and methodology for measuring accuracy differed considerably from those of Fan et al. (they did not report on quantitative differences between planned and actual screw directions), a comparison of the results of the two studies presents challenges [31]. Nevertheless, it can be concluded that again 3DPG evidences a high degree of accuracy and that the finding of the current study validates with more confidence that the accuracy of screw insertion using 3DPG is similar and non-inferior to that of CAS.

4.1. Implications of the Study's Findings

In light of the findings of this study, 3DPG can be considered to be an effective and accurate alternative navigational technology relative to CAS for cervical and thoracic spine fixation. It is important to point out that the results obtained using 3DPG cannot be pre-guaranteed when implementing the same technique and that our surgical teams underwent a learning curve, performing several cadaveric surgeries that served as training sessions. Furthermore, our comprehensive point-of-care 3D planning and printing facility has evolved over time, and we have acquired sufficient professional knowledge and competent staff with extensive training, enabling us to guarantee high-quality performance standards in full compliance with the EU medical device regulation (EU 2017/745). Centers that lack these facilities should be made aware of the high-quality standards that are required, or they should find suitable commercial partners for VSP and PSI design. However, given the technology's novelty, its commercial availability is currently limited.

Although 3D technology has great potential, the technique is not suitable for all cases. This particularly applies for trauma cases that require immediate fixation surgery. Since the here described technology needs pre-planning, manufacturing and sterilization of 3D-printed instrumentation, the whole process does at minimum require 3–4 days. Additionally, for minimal invasive approaches the current 3D technology is not yet suitable. However, minimal invasive screw insertion gains increased popularity in order to minimize tissue trauma. Three-dimensional printed guides for minimal invasive approaches remains largely and unexplored area. There are however few examples of which the SpineBox system is the most well-known [35]. Further studies are needed in this area to compare these new approaches with CAS technology.

4.2. Study Limitations

At our center, the CAS system was used in combination with a 3D fluoroscopy C-arm capable of acquiring an intraoperative cone beam CT scan. Current state-of-the-art CAS systems are, however, often installed with the newer O-arms, which potentially provide enhanced image quality. Although both systems offer high levels of accuracy, there is some evidence that the use of O-arms with CAS improves the level of accuracy [36]. Therefore, our results are not generalizable for all CAS set-ups. Consequently, future studies that entail direct comparisons of 3DPG and O-arm-equipped CAS are warranted.

Within current 3D fluoroscopy CAS systems, the screw trajectory is defined 'on the spot', and not according to a predefined screw plan. Therefore, in the present study, we could not measure the accuracy of CAS accuracy with respect to a preoperative plan;

instead, we measured its accuracy using the saved, intraoperative acquired trajectories and CT image data. It is possible that the surgeon considered the trajectory associated with the acquired hole to be sufficient but not optimal. If accuracy is defined according to the extent of deviation from the most optimal trajectory, the study could entail a slight overestimation of the actual accuracy of CAS. This again exposes the major advantage of 3DPG; the optimal trajectory can be selected and considered preoperatively instead of being defined during the time-constrained and intensive period of surgery.

A consideration of more clinical variables, such as infection rates, intraoperative blood loss, duration of the operation, and radiation dosage, was beyond the scope of the current study design. Additionally, for analyzing subgroups with different screw techniques (lateral mass or pedicle) the study was insufficiently powered. Consequently, these variables were not included in the comparison of the two techniques. Therefore, prospective RCTs with larger sample sizes are still required for a comprehensive assessment of these two techniques. It is likely that higher-powered clinical trials are necessary to validate our findings with a higher degree of confidence and to evaluate whether the inclusion of other clinical parameters, such as surgery time (total/per screw), support the use of one or the other technique.

Our analysis of both end points was performed on a per-protocol basis. During the study, there was a drop out of 3 patients due to data loss, which should be prevented in future studies by multiple copies or cloud storage. In addition, some of vertebral levels that we had planned to include in the fusion were not instrumented in cases entailing a sufficient amount of fixation. Because these screws were not inserted, they could not be evaluated, making an intention-to-treat analysis impossible to perform. Therefore, only planned screws that were actually in situ and visible as postoperative image data were included in the analysis. Furthermore, in our opinion, an intention-to-treat analysis was not appropriate for the current study design because randomization pertained to the level of patient side rather than to patients. An intension-to-treat analysis would, therefore, only be necessary when for example the assigned sided were revered, which is something that did not occur in this study.

Within-patient clustering was not considered in this study. In the future, variance and thus confidence intervals need to be inflated to account for the effect of within-patient clustering for two main reasons. Firstly, because screws within patients are more likely to resemble each other than screws across different patients (violating the independence assumption) and secondly because treatment is assigned on the level of patient side, not on the level of the screw. Therefore, to accurately reflect dependencies in the data, cluster-randomized design (whereby patients are the clusters) will be used to appropriately power future studies.

5. Conclusions

Although the benefits of 3DPG and its accuracy have been repeatedly demonstrated, this is the first randomized controlled study that compares 3DPG with CAS. The results of this RCT indicate that the accuracy of spinal screw insertion using 3DPG is similar and non-inferior to that obtained with CAS. Future higher powered comparative studies should focus on studying specific subgroups of vertebral levels that have the potential to demonstrate superiority.

Author Contributions: Conceptualization, P.A.J.P., J.M.A.K., D.L.M.O., R.A.V., G.R., M.H.C., J.K. and R.J.M.G.; data curation, P.A.J.P. and J.M.A.K.; formal analysis, P.A.J.P., K.T. and J.M.A.K.; investigation, P.A.J.P., J.M.A.K., K.T., D.L.M.O., R.A.V., G.R., M.H.C., J.K. and R.J.M.G.; methodology, P.A.J.P., J.M.A.K., J.K. and R.J.M.G.; project administration, P.A.J.P.; resources, P.A.J.P. and J.K.; software, P.A.J.P. and J.K.; supervision, J.M.A.K., J.K. and R.J.M.G.; validation, P.A.J.P. and J.K.; visualization, P.A.J.P.; writing—original draft, P.A.J.P.; writing—review and editing, J.M.A.K., K.T., D.L.M.O., R.A.V., G.R., M.H.C., J.K. and R.J.M.G. All authors have read and agreed to the published version of the manuscript.

Funding: This research received no external funding.

Institutional Review Board Statement: The study was conducted in accordance with the Declaration of Helsinki and approved by the Institutional Review Board (or Ethics Committee) of University Medical Center Groningen (ref. no. M19.229543 and date of approval 3-4-2019).

Informed Consent Statement: Informed consent was obtained from all subjects involved in the study. Written informed consent has been obtained from the patients to publish this paper.

Data Availability Statement: The authors declare that the data supporting the findings of this study are available within the paper.

Acknowledgments: We thank Diane Steenks for her administrative support in executing this study.

Conflicts of Interest: The authors declare no conflict of interest.

References

1. Esses, S.I.; Sachs, B.L.; Dreyzin, V. Complications associated with the technique of pedicle screw fixation. A selected survey of ABS members. *Spine* **1993**, *18*, 2231–2238. [CrossRef]
2. Gertzbein, S.D.; Robbins, S.E. Accuracy of pedicular screw placement in vivo. *Spine* **1990**, *15*, 11–14. [CrossRef] [PubMed]
3. Gaines, R.W., Jr. The use of pedicle-screw internal fixation for the operative treatment of spinal disorders. *J. Bone Jt. Surg. Am.* **2000**, *82*, 1458. [CrossRef] [PubMed]
4. Blumenthal, S.; Gill, K. Complications of the Wiltse Pedicle Screw Fixation System. *Spine* **1993**, *18*, 1867–1871. [CrossRef] [PubMed]
5. Liljenqvist, U.R.; Halm, H.F.H.; Link, T.M. Pedicle screw instrumentation of the thoracic spine in idiopathic scoliosis. *Spine* **1997**, *22*, 2239–2245. [CrossRef] [PubMed]
6. Vaccaro, A.R.; Rizzolo, S.J.; Balderston, R.A.; Allardyce, T.J.; Garfin, S.R.; Dolinskas, C.; An, H.S. Placement of pedicle screws in the thoracic spine. Part II: An anatomical and radiographic assessment. *J. Bone Jt. Surg. Am.* **1995**, *77*, 1200–1206. [CrossRef] [PubMed]
7. Luther, N.; Iorgulescu, J.B.; Geannette, C.; Gebhard, H.; Saleh, T.; Tsiouris, A.J.; Härtl, R. Comparison of navigated versus non-navigated pedicle screw placement in 260 patients and 1434 screws. *J. Spinal Disord. Tech.* **2015**, *28*, E298–E303. [CrossRef]
8. Yu, X.; Xu, L.; Bi, L.Y. Spinal navigation with intra-operative 3D-imaging modality in lumbar pedicle screw fixation. *Zhonghua Yi Xue Za Zhi* **2008**, *88*, 1905–1908.
9. Austin, M.S.; Vaccaro, A.R.; Brislin, B.; Nachwalter, R.; Hilibrand, A.S.; Albert, T.J. Image-guided spine surgery: A cadaver study comparing conventional open laminoforaminotomy and two image-guided techniques for pedicle screw placement in posterolateral fusion and nonfusion models. *Spine* **2002**, *27*, 2503–2508. [CrossRef]
10. Ishikawa, Y.; Kanemura, T.; Yoshida, G.; Ito, Z.; Muramoto, A.; Ohno, S. Clinical accuracy of three-dimensional fluoroscopy-based computer-assisted cervical pedicle screw placement: A retrospective comparative study of conventional versus computer-assisted cervical pedicle screw placement. *J. Neurosurg. Spine* **2010**, *13*, 606–611. [CrossRef]
11. Schepers, R.H.; Raghoebar, G.M.; Vissink, A.; Stenekes, M.W.; Kraeima, J.; Roodenburg, J.L.; Reintsema, H.; Witjes, M.J. Accuracy of fibula reconstruction using patient-specific CAD/CAM reconstruction plates and dental implants: A new modality for functional reconstruction of mandibular defects. *J. Cranio-Maxillofac. Surg.* **2015**, *43*, 649–657. [CrossRef] [PubMed]
12. Lu, S.; Xu, Y.Q.; Chen, G.P.; Zhang, Y.Z.; Lu, D.; Chen, Y.B.; Shi, J.H.; Xu, X.M. Efficacy and accuracy of a novel rapid prototyping drill template for cervical pedicle screw placement. *Comput. Aided Surg.* **2011**, *16*, 240–248. [CrossRef] [PubMed]
13. Ma, T.; Xu, Y.Q.; Cheng, Y.B.; Jiang, M.Y.; Xu, X.M.; Xie, L.; Lu, S. A novel computer-assisted drill guide template for thoracic pedicle screw placement: A cadaveric study. *Arch. Orthop. Trauma Surg.* **2012**, *132*, 65–72. [CrossRef] [PubMed]
14. Bundoc, R.C.; Delgado, G.D.G.; Grozman, S.A.M. A novel patient-specific drill guide template for pedicle screw insertion into the subaxial cervical spine utilizing stereolithographic modelling: An in vitro study. *Asian Spine J.* **2017**, *11*, 4–14. [CrossRef] [PubMed]
15. Zhang, G.; Yu, Z.; Chen, X.; Chen, X.; Wu, C.; Lin, Y.; Huang, W.; Lin, H. Accurate placement of cervical pedicle screws using 3D-printed navigational templates. *Orthopade* **2018**, *47*, 428–436. [CrossRef]
16. Yu, Z.; Zhang, G.; Chen, X.; Chen, X.; Wu, C.; Lin, Y.; Huang, W.; Lin, H. Application of a novel 3D drill template for cervical pedicle screw tunnel design: A cadaveric study. *Eur. Spine J.* **2017**, *26*, 2348–2356. [CrossRef]
17. Pijpker, P.A.J.; Kraeima, J.; Witjes, M.J.H.; Oterdoom, D.L.M.; Coppes, M.H.; Groen, R.J.M.; Kuijlen, J.M.A. Accuracy Assessment of Pedicle and Lateral Mass Screw Insertion Assisted by Customized 3D-Printed Drill Guides: A Human Cadaver Study. *Oper. Neurosurg.* **2019**, *16*, 94–102. [CrossRef]
18. Owen, B.; Christensen, G.; Reinhardt, J.; Ryken, T. Rapid prototype patient-specific drill template for cervical pedicle screw placement. *Comput. Aided Surg.* **2007**, *12*, 303–308. [CrossRef]
19. Lu, S.; Xu, Y.Q.; Lu, W.W.; Ni, G.X.; Li, Y.B.; Shi, J.H.; Li, D.P.; Chen, G.P.; Chen, Y.B.; Zhang, Y.Z. A novel patient-specific navigational template for cervical pedicle screw placement. *Spine* **2009**, *34*, E959–E966. [CrossRef]

20. Kim, S.B.; Won, Y.; Yoo, H.J.; Sin, L.J.; Rhee, J.M.; Lee, S.W.; Lee, G.S. Unilateral Spinous Process Noncovering Hook Type Patient-specific Drill Template for Thoracic Pedicle Screw Fixation. *Spine* **2017**, *42*, E1050–E1057. [CrossRef]
21. Kaneyama, S.; Sugawara, T.; Sumi, M. Safe and accurate midcervical pedicle screw insertion procedure with the patient-specific screw guide template system. *Spine* **2015**, *40*, E341–E348. [CrossRef]
22. Takemoto, M.; Fujibayashi, S.; Ota, E.; Otsuki, B. Additive-manufactured patient-specific titanium templates for thoracic pedicle screw placement: Novel design with reduced contact area. *Eur. Spine J.* **2016**, *25*, 1698–1705. [CrossRef] [PubMed]
23. Pijpker, P.A.J.; Kraeima, J.; Witjes, M.J.H.; Oterdoom, D.L.M.; Vergeer, R.A.; Coppes, M.H.; Groen, R.J.M.; Kuijlen, J.M.A. Accuracy of Patient-Specific 3D-Printed Drill Guides for Pedicle and Lateral Mass Screw Insertion: An Analysis of 76 Cervical and Thoracic Screw Trajectories. *Spine* **2021**, *46*, 160–168. [CrossRef] [PubMed]
24. Lu, S.; Zhang, Y.Z.; Wang, Z.; Shi, J.H.; Chen, Y.B.; Xu, X.M.; Xu, Y.Q. Accuracy and efficacy of thoracic pedicle screws in scoliosis with patient-specific drill template. *Med. Biol. Eng. Comput.* **2012**, *50*, 751–758. [CrossRef]
25. Liu, K.; Zhang, Q.; Li, X.; Zhao, C.; Quan, X.; Zhao, R.; Chen, Z.; Li, Y. Preliminary application of a multi-level 3D printing drill guide template for pedicle screw placement in severe and rigid scoliosis. *Eur. Spine J.* **2017**, *26*, 1684–1689. [CrossRef] [PubMed]
26. Lu, S.; Xu, Y.Q.; Zhang, Y.Z.; Xie, L.; Guo, H.; Li, D.P. A novel computer-assisted drill guide template for placement of C_2 laminar screws. *Eur. Spine J.* **2009**, *18*, 1379–1385. [CrossRef]
27. Goffin, J.; Van Brussel, K.; Martens, K. Three-Dimensional Computed Tomography-Based, Personalized Drill Guide for Posterior Cervical Stabilization at C1–C2. *Spine* **2001**, *26*, 1343–1347. [CrossRef]
28. Cecchinato, R.; Berjano, P.; Zerbi, A.; Damilano, M.; Redaelli, A.; Lamartina, C. Pedicle screw insertion with patient-specific 3D-printed guides based on low-dose CT scan is more accurate than free-hand technique in spine deformity patients: A prospective, randomized clinical trial. *Eur. Spine J.* **2019**, *28*, 1712–1723. [CrossRef]
29. Feng, S.; Lin, J.; Su, N.; Meng, H.; Yang, Y.; Fei, Q. 3-Dimensional printing templates guiding versus free hand technique for cervical lateral mass screw fixation: A prospective study. *J. Clin. Neurosci. Off. J. Neurosurg. Soc. Australas.* **2020**, *78*, 252–258. [CrossRef]
30. Fan, Y.; Du, J.-P.; Wu, Q.-N.; Zhang, J.-N.; Hao, D.-J. Accuracy of a patient-specific template for pedicle screw placement compared with a conventional method: A meta-analysis. *Arch. Orthop. Trauma Surg.* **2017**, *137*, 1641–1649. [CrossRef]
31. Fan, Y.; Du, J.; Zhang, J.; Liu, S.; Xue, X.; Huang, Y.; Zhang, J.; Hao, D. Comparison of Accuracy of Pedicle Screw Insertion Among 4 Guided Technologies in Spine Surgery. *Med. Sci. Monit. Int. Med. J. Exp. Clin. Res.* **2017**, *23*, 5960–5968. [CrossRef] [PubMed]
32. Uneri, A.; De Silva, T.; Stayman, J.W.; Kleinszig, G.; Vogt, S.; Khanna, A.J.; Gokaslan, Z.L.; Wolinsky, J.-P.; Siewerdsen, J.H. Known-component 3D-2D registration for quality assurance of spine surgery pedicle screw placement. *Phys. Med. Biol.* **2015**, *60*, 8007–8024. [CrossRef] [PubMed]
33. Rampersaud, Y.R.; Simon, D.A.; Foley, K.T. Accuracy requirements for image-guided spinal pedicle screw placement. *Spine* **2001**, *26*, 352–359. [CrossRef] [PubMed]
34. Ishikawa, Y.; Kanemura, T.; Yoshida, G.; Matsumoto, A.; Ito, Z.; Tauchi, R.; Muramoto, A.; Ohno, S.; Nishimura, Y. Intraoperative, full-rotation, three-dimensional image (O-arm)-based navigation system for cervical pedicle screw insertion. *J. Neurosurg. Spine* **2011**, *15*, 472–478. [CrossRef] [PubMed]
35. Thayaparan, G.K.; Owbridge, M.G.; Linden, M.; Thompson, R.G.; Lewis, P.M.; D'Urso, P.S. Measuring the performance of patient-specific solutions for minimally invasive transforaminal lumbar interbody fusion surgery. *J. Clin. Neurosci.* **2020**, *71*, 43–50. [CrossRef] [PubMed]
36. Banat, M.; Wach, J.; Salemdawod, A.; Bahna, M.; Scorzin, J.; Vatter, H. The Role of Intraoperative Image Guidance Systems (Three-Dimensional C-arm versus O-arm) in Spinal Surgery: Results of a Single-Center Study. *World Neurosurg.* **2021**, *146*, e817–e821. [CrossRef]

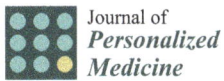

Article

Does a Customized 3D Printing Plate Based on Virtual Reduction Facilitate the Restoration of Original Anatomy in Fractures?

Seung-Han Shin [1], Moo-Sub Kim [2], Do-Kun Yoon [2], Jae-Jin Lee [2] and Yang-Guk Chung [1,*]

1. Department of Orthopedic Surgery, Seoul St. Mary's Hospital, College of Medicine, The Catholic University of Korea, Seoul 06591, Korea; tumorshin@gmail.com
2. Industrial R&D Center, KAVILAB Co., Ltd., Seoul 06693, Korea; mskim@kavilab.ai (M.-S.K.); dbsehrns@naver.com (D.-K.Y.); hiiamjjinli@gmail.com (J.-J.L.)
* Correspondence: ygchung@catholic.ac.kr

Abstract: The purpose of this study was to evaluate the restoration of original anatomy after fixation of sawbone fractures using case-specific 3D printing plates based on virtual reduction (VR). Three-dimensional models of 28 tibia sawbones with cortical marking holes were obtained. The sawbones were fractured at various locations of the shaft and 3D models were obtained. The fractured models were reduced virtually and customized non-locking metal plates that fit the reduced model were produced via 3D printing. The fractured sawbones were actually fixed to the customized plate with nonlocking screws and 3D models were generated. With the proximal fragments of the 3D models overlapped, the changes in length, 3D angulation, and rotation of the distal fragment were evaluated. Compared to the intact model (IN), the virtual reduction model (VR) and the actual fixation model (AF) showed no significant differences in length. Compared to the IN, the VR and the AF had mean 3D angulations of 0.39° and 0.64°, respectively. Compared to the IN model, the VR and the AF showed mean rotations of 0.89° and 1.51°, respectively. A customized plate based on VR facilitates the restoration of near-original anatomy in fractures of tibial sawbone shaft.

Keywords: fracture; virtual reduction; 3D printing; patient-specific customized plate

Citation: Shin, S.-H.; Kim, M.-S.; Yoon, D.-K.; Lee, J.-J.; Chung, Y.-G. Does a Customized 3D Printing Plate Based on Virtual Reduction Facilitate the Restoration of Original Anatomy in Fractures? *J. Pers. Med.* **2022**, *12*, 927. https://doi.org/10.3390/jpm12060927

Academic Editors: Joep Kraeima, Sebastiaan de Visscher and Max J.H. Witjes

Received: 20 May 2022
Accepted: 30 May 2022
Published: 2 June 2022

Publisher's Note: MDPI stays neutral with regard to jurisdictional claims in published maps and institutional affiliations.

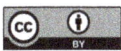

Copyright: © 2022 by the authors. Licensee MDPI, Basel, Switzerland. This article is an open access article distributed under the terms and conditions of the Creative Commons Attribution (CC BY) license (https://creativecommons.org/licenses/by/4.0/).

1. Introduction

Fractures are a relatively common injury. In 2019, there were 178 million new fractures worldwide (increased by 33.4% since 1990) and the age-standardized rate of fractures was 2296.2 per 100,000 population [1]. Surgical treatment of fractures has increased along with the increase in the demand for normal functional recovery via anatomical reduction [2–4].

Since Hansmann first reported fracture fixation using plate and screws in 1886, plate osteosynthesis has become the standard for fracture surgeries, especially for articular and metaphyseal fractures and some diaphyseal fractures such as those involving the forearm [5]. Fracture plates have evolved over time, and currently anatomically pre-contoured locking plates are widely used [6,7].

However, despite the evolution of the plates, intraoperative anatomical fixation still entails manual reduction of the fracture, followed by plate contouring because a single anatomical plate does not fit all the patients. Patient-specific fracture plates may overcome such inconvenience but they are still to be developed, although various patient-specific treatments employing three-dimensional (3D) printing technology have recently been used. The lack of a model for case-specific plate design is one of the primary hurdles in this area.

In this study, we used the virtual reduction (VR) of a fracture as the basis for designing customized plates. The purpose of this study was to evaluate the restoration of original anatomy after the actual fixation of sawbone fractures using 3D printed plates based on VR.

2. Materials and Methods

2.1. Experimental Procedures

A total of 28 tibial sawbones (ORTHObones model W19122, W19126, W19129, and W19131, size 15.4 in × 31.9 in × 2.8 in, weight 0.35 kg, 3B Scientific, Hamburg, Germany) were used, and the overall experimental flow is depicted in Figure 1. In each sawbone, cortical marking holes were drilled to consistently localize the same measurement points on the 3D models obtained by multiple scanning. Three cortical marking holes were drilled in the same proximal axial plane and another three holes were drilled in the same distal axial plane using a customized jig. Each one of the three holes was located in the mid-sagittal plane of the tibia. Following computed tomography (CT), 3D models of the sawbones were obtained using MIMICS software (Ver 21.0, Materialise, Leuven, Belgium); these models were categorized as intact (IN). Using this software, the 3D coordinates of the center of each marking hole were automatically calculated so that subsequent measurements could be performed without observer bias.

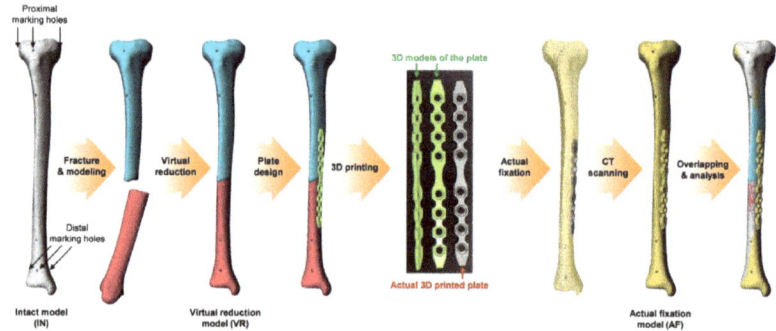

Figure 1. Overall experimental flow. Three-dimensional, (3D).

The sawbones were fractured at various longitudinal locations of the shaft (Figure 2A), and 3D models were obtained after CT scan. The fractured models were reduced virtually using Metasequoia 4 software (Ver 4.7.0, Tetraface, Tokyo, Japan); these models were grouped under the virtual reduction (VR) category.

Using the same software, a case-specific fracture fixation plate with four screw holes for proximal fragment and four screw holes for distal fragment was designed to fit the medial surface of each VR model. The contact surface (with bone) of the plate was designed according to the Boolean function in Metasequoia 4 to ensure perfect contact between the bone surface and the plate. The plates were then fabricated using a powder bed fusion type 3D printer (DMP 350, 3D Systems, SC) and titanium powder (grade 23 Ti-6Al-4V alloy). Post-processing consisted of removal of the supporter, surface finishing using a hand piece, and blasting with ceramic microbead. The dimensions of the plates were 149.5 ± 1 mm in length, 12 ± 0.1 mm in width, and 2.5 ± 0.1 mm in thickness. The actual fractured sawbones were reduced and fixed to the plate with nonlocking screws to ensure complete contact of the fragments with the customized plate (Figure 2B). Three-dimensional models of the fixed sawbones obtained after CT scan were grouped under the actual fixation (AF) category.

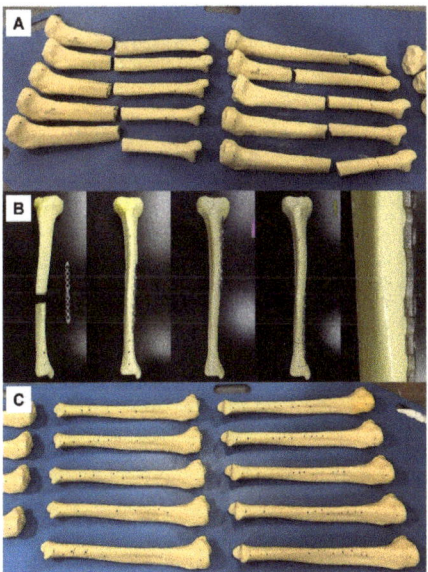

Figure 2. (**A**) Tibial sawbones fractured at various longitudinal locations of the shaft, prior to CT scan. (**B**) Sawbones and customized plates prior to fixation (left image in row), fixed at various locations (middle three images in row), and enlarged at the fracture site (right image in row). (**C**) Tibial sawbones actually fixed with a customized plate based on virtual reduction, prior to CT scan.

2.2. Evaluation of the Alignment

To evaluate the alignment after VR and AF, the IN, VR, and AF models of each sawbone were overlapped virtually in 3D space while ensuring the same position of the proximal fragments of each model (Figure 3). Sagittal, coronal, and axial planes were set to fit the shape of the tibia. The alignment was evaluated based on three parameters: length of the model, angulation of the distal fragment, and rotation of the distal fragment.

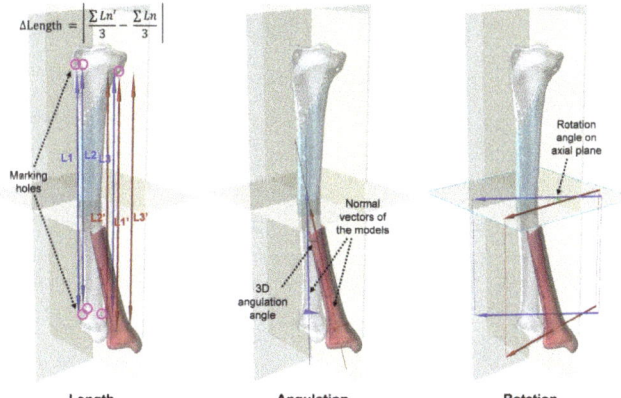

Figure 3. Evaluation of the alignment with the proximal fragment of the models overlapped: length (the mean distance between marking holes in longitudinal axis), angulation (3D angle between normal vectors of the distal fragments), and rotation (the angle between the axial plane projections of the vectors passing through two of the three distal marking holes).

The length of each model was defined as the average distance in the longitudinal direction between the centers of the marking holes proximal 3 and distal 3. The lengths of the IN, VR, and AF models were compared. The differences in the length of VR compared to that of IN and the length of AF compared to that of IN were also measured. The angulation of the distal fragment was defined as the 3D angle between the normal vector of the distal fragment of IN and that of VR or AF. The normal vector of the distal fragment was obtained from the plane containing the centers of three distal marking holes. The degree of angulation for VR and AF was compared. The rotation of the distal fragment was defined as the angle between the axial plane projection of the vector passing through two of the centers of the three distal marking holes of IN and that of VR or AF. The degrees of rotation for VR and AF were also calculated and compared.

2.3. Statistical Analysis

Statistical analyses were conducted using Statistics and Machine Learning Toolbox on MATLAB (R2021b, MathWorks, Natick, MA, USA). Descriptive statistics are presented as mean (M) and standard variation (SD). The significance of the differences in the mean values of each evaluated parameter was analyzed via paired t-tests after verifying the normality of the data distribution. The significance level was set at $p < 0.05$.

3. Results

The mean lengths of the IN, VR, and AF models were 329.22 mm (SD, 2.92 mm; range, 323.50–336.21 mm), 329.15 mm (SD, 2.88 mm; range, 323.66–336.03 mm), and 329.51 mm (SD, 2.82 mm; range, 324.05–335.92 mm), respectively (Figure 4A). There were no significant differences in length between any two of the three models ($p > 0.05$). The mean length difference (either lengthening or shortening) of VR relative to IN was 0.17 mm (SD, 0.14 mm; range, 0–0.81 mm), which was significantly greater than that of AF relative to IN (0.36 mm, SD, 0.29 mm; range, 0–1.32 mm) ($p = 0.0001$) (Figure 4B).

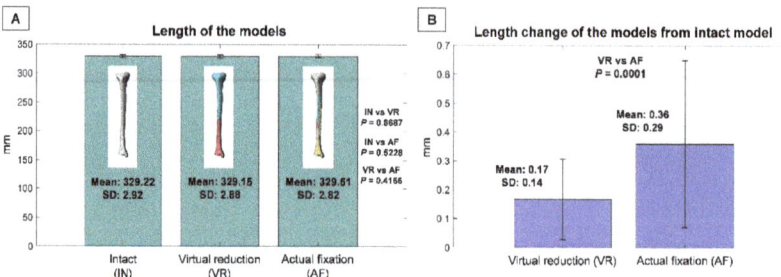

Figure 4. (**A**) Lengths of intact (IN), virtual reduction (VR), and actual fixation (AF) models. (**B**) Length variation of VR compared to IN and that of AF compared to IN. Standard deviation, (SD).

The mean angulation of VR relative to IN was 0.39° (SD, 0.28°; range, 0–0.92°), which was not significantly different from the mean angulation of AF relative to IN (0.64°, SD, 0.65°; range, 0–3.01°) ($p = 0.0611$) (Figure 5). The mean rotation of VR relative to IN was 0.89° (SD, 0.76°; range, 0.09–3.34°), which was not significantly different from that of AF relative to IN (1.51°, SD, 1.87°; range, 0–9.54°) ($p = 0.1138$) (Figure 6).

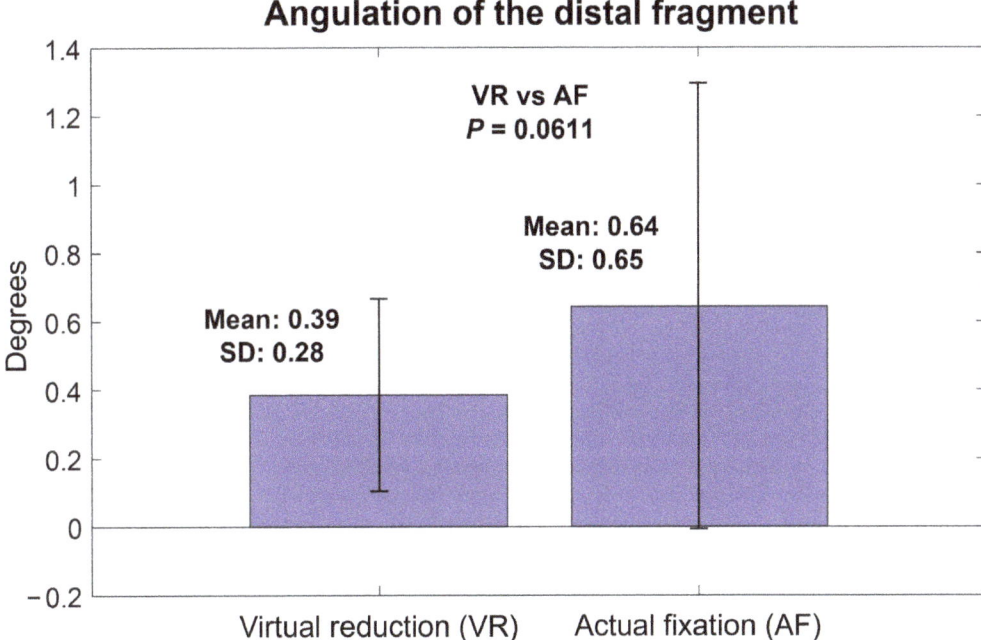

Figure 5. Angulation of virtual reduction and actual fixation models relative to intact models.

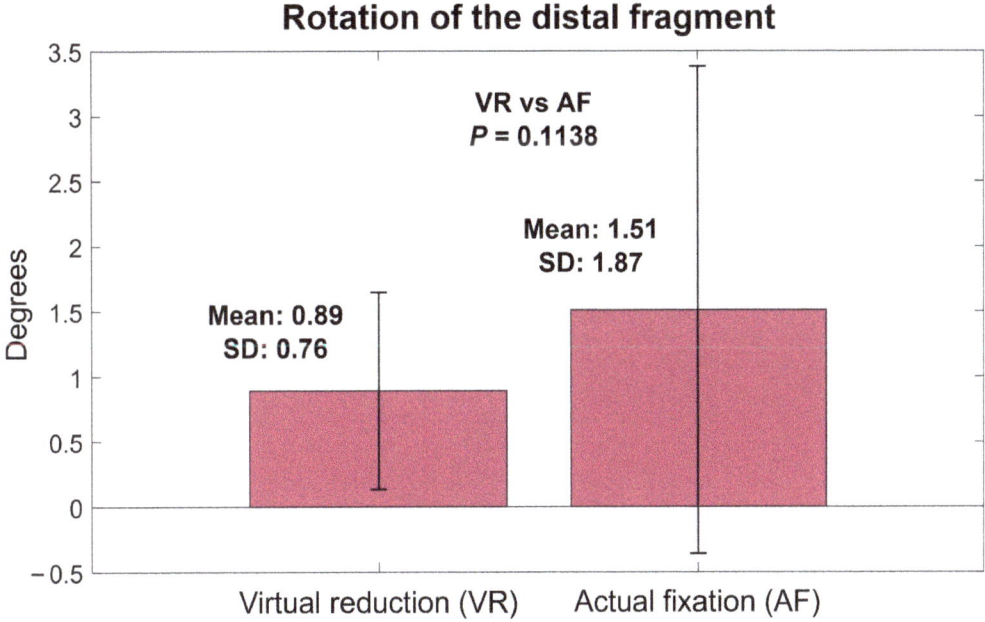

Figure 6. Rotation of virtual reduction and actual fixation models relative to intact models.

4. Discussion

The principal finding of the current study is that a fractured bone can be reduced to near its original anatomy with a customized plate based on virtual reduction. The tibia was chosen for this study because it has sufficient length and width on which to place the marking holes far from each other so that the alignment could be measured accurately. The fracture was made at various longitudinal locations of the tibial shaft to simulate various innate anatomy features (curvatures and twists on the surface) at the fracture site. The acceptable range of fracture reduction alignment is generally evaluated by length, angulation, and rotation [8,9]. For a tibia fracture, 10–20 mm shortening, 5–10° angulation, and 10–20° rotation are considered to be acceptable [10]. Tibial malunion occurs in 3–50% of conservative treatment and up to 20% of surgical fixation [10]. Although plate osteosynthesis has the lowest malunion rate for tibial fractures [11–13], the malunion rate reaches up to 8.3% even after tibial plating [14], and midshaft fractures do not have a lower malunion rate than distal fractures [15]. The mean angulation after tibial plating reaches up to 2.6–3.1° even on a single coronal plane [16,17]. In our results, both VR and AF showed minor mean changes in length (0.17 and 0.36 mm), angulation (0.39 and 0.64°), and rotation (0.89 and 1.51°) compared to the pre-fracture condition. These results suggest that the alignment effect of the VR-based plate itself is excellent, although further studies are needed to investigate whether the final alignment will equal the alignment immediately after fixation in clinical practice.

At present, fracture surgery using a metal plate involves manual reduction of the fragments followed by manual contouring of the plate to fit the reduced bone. Sometimes the manual reduction itself is difficult and may require alignment verification with intraoperative radiographs because the operator can only see the exposed part of the bone. Even with successful reduction, repeated manual bending and twisting of the plate is necessary to fit the plate to the reduced bone. Although contemporary locking plates do not need to fit to the bone for stability [18,19], at least some manual contouring is still necessary, even for anatomical plates, to install the plate and screws in the right position and prevent plate protrusion or irritation. These procedures require additional surgical time, effort, and equipment. The outcomes of the fixation may vary depending on the operator's experience or know-how. Further, there are cases in which a plate does not fit the bone despite bending and twisting, or an important fragment cannot be purchased because the screw holes are limited to certain fixed locations.

To address these limitations, studies have utilized 3D printing technology in fracture surgeries. The application of 3D printing in fractures varies widely from 3D modeling for screw fixation to customized casting [20,21]. The existing works on 3D printing fracture plates can be largely divided into tactile modeling and mirroring of the normal contralateral bone. Recent reports of tactile modeling techniques have involved real-size 3D printing of the fractured bone for pre-practicing of the surgery and pre-contouring of the plate [22–24]. Although tactile modeling reduces intraoperative time, blood loss, and fluoroscopies [25], the overall procedure still entails manual reduction of the tactile model and bending and twisting of the plate by the operator.

Meanwhile, the other type of approach utilizes mirroring of the normal contralateral bone. Various authors have used mirrored models to pre-contour a ready-made plate and achieved good outcomes [26–28]. A recent study reported 3D printed case-specific pelvic fracture plates based on a mirrored 3D model of the contralateral pelvis [29]. When using such a strategy, manual pre-reduction of the fracture is not necessary to pre-contour the plate. However, in practice, there are cases in which a normal contralateral image is not available, such as cases involving bilateral fractures or when the patent refuses to undergo an additional CT of the uninjured other side. The difference between right and left bones may also be problematic and may lead to malalignment after reduction or protrusion of the plate. A poorly-fitting 3D printed plate may be especially problematic because it is still difficult to ensure both strength and ductility of 3D printed metals [30,31] and bending of the 3D printed plate may result in fracture.

However, in this study, we used a virtually reduced model as the basis of each case-specific fracture plate and thus achieved near-original alignment. Our results suggest that the virtually reduced bone represents an excellent model for designing case-specific fracture plates. The VR has advantages over intraoperative manual reduction in which the operator only visualizes the exposed area of the bone or has to perform fluoroscopy. Further, compared to the mirror method, the VR does not result in errors caused by differences between right and left bones, and it does not increase the cost or radiation exposure during contralateral imaging.

In addition to the excellent fit, the VR-based customized plate has an advantage in which the plate itself can guide fracture reduction intraoperatively. Because the plate is designed to fit the reduced model, the operator can both reduce the fracture and determine the alignment by attaching the bone fragments to the plate. In conventional fracture fixation, the operator manually reduces the bone, determines the alignment, and temporarily clamps the fragments to hold the reduction. Then a plate is placed on the surface of the bone, and is bent and twisted accordingly. These procedures may require considerable amounts of intraoperative time and effort. In addition, sometimes the clamp holding the reduction hinders the attachment of the plate onto the bone to determine the fit. By contrast, our method involved screwing the fragments to the plate with nonlocking screws to ensure complete contact. The procedure was simpler and restored almost original anatomy of the fractured sawbones. This may allow less-experienced surgeons to operate easily and quickly, reduce radiation exposure and need for related equipment, and prevent plate-related complications such as plate protrusion or irritation. In addition, good contact between the bone and the plate may strengthen the fixation and facilitate better alignment in minimally invasive plate osteosynthesis.

However, the VR-based plate is not completely free from performance-related errors, in that the mean length of VR model was shorter than that of IN model, and in that the length difference of AF was significantly greater than that of VR. In some cases, the task performer for the VR had to let the virtual fragment slightly intrude into the other virtual fragment to obtain better overall alignment. This made the mean length of the VR model shorter, although this difference was not statistically significant. The significantly greater length difference of AF can be attributed to the surgical technique. The angulation and rotation were also greater in AF than in VR, although this difference was also not statistically significant. For example, compression across the fracture site due to eccentric placement of the screws resulted in a slight gap between the far cortices at the fracture site (Figure 2). Although the overall final alignment was excellent in our study, there is room for achieving even better alignment with the additional use of appropriate techniques such as centering the screws in the holes while using the customized plate. Designing the plate slightly concave to the bone to allow compression across the fracture site may also improve the final alignment. Further studies are needed to investigate these possibilities.

The current study has limitations. First, no comparisons were performed with conventional or mirroring-based plates. However, the final alignment parameters were adequate to ensure fracture surgeries. Second, a single type of sawbone was used, and relatively simple fractures were simulated. Although we simulated the individuality of each bone shape and fracture type by making the fractures at different longitudinal locations, additional studies involving various bones and complex fractures are needed to further confirm the reliability of VR. Third, this study was an experimental study, and it did not take into account in vivo conditions such as the soft tissue or the bone quality. In practice, the final alignment of the bone can be affected by soft tissue tension or low bone density. In vivo evaluations based on the present work are necessary to further investigate the clinical relevance of the customized fracture plates. However, in practice, the original anatomy is missing when fracture patients visit a clinic, which means there is a need for an experimental study to accurately evaluate the aligning effect of the customized plate. For such a study, we believe that a sawbone experiment is the best because, in an in vivo experiment, the soft tissue or the bone quality may confound the aligning effect of the customized plate itself. Lastly, before our method can be actually applied in fracture surgeries, further studies are needed to reduce the time needed for image engineering and manufacturing, and to ensure the mechanical properties of the customized plates.

In conclusion, a customized plate based on VR facilitates the restoration of near-original anatomy in fractures of tibial sawbone shaft. Besides the excellent fit, the plate itself can guide the alignment of fracture reduction. The use of a VR model as the basis of implant design may facilitate the application of 3D printing technology in personalized fracture surgeries.

Author Contributions: Conceptualization, S.-H.S. and Y.-G.C.; methodology, S.-H.S.; software, M.-S.K. and D.-K.Y.; validation, S.-H.S. and Y.-G.C.; formal analysis, M.-S.K. and D.-K.Y.; investigation, S.-H.S., M.-S.K., D.-K.Y. and J.-J.L.; resources, J.-J.L.; data curation, M.-S.K. and D.-K.Y.; writing—original draft preparation, S.-H.S.; writing—review and editing, Y.-G.C.; visualization, D.-K.Y.; supervision, Y.-G.C.; funding acquisition, S.-H.S. and Y.-G.C. All authors have read and agreed to the published version of the manuscript.

Funding: This study was supported by the Research Fund of Seoul St. Mary's Hospital, The Catholic University of Korea, the National Research Foundation of Korea (NRF) grant funded by the Korea government (MSIT) (No. 2019R1G1A1100754), and the Technology Innovation Program (No. 20000397, Development of 2Track Customized 3D Printing Implant Manufacturing and Commercializing Techniques for Complex Bone Fractures) funded by the Ministry of Trade, Industry & Energy (MOTIE, Korea). The funding sources did not play a role in the investigation.

Institutional Review Board Statement: Not applicable.

Informed Consent Statement: Not applicable.

Data Availability Statement: The data presented in this study are available on request from the corresponding author.

Conflicts of Interest: The authors declare no conflict of interest.

References

1. GBD 2019 Fracture Collaborators. Global, regional, and national burden of bone fractures in 204 countries and territories, 1990-2019: A systematic analysis from the Global Burden of Disease Study 2019. *Lancet Healthy Longev.* **2021**, *2*, e580–e592. [CrossRef]
2. Chung, K.C.; Shauver, M.J.; Birkmeyer, J.D. Trends in the United States in the treatment of distal radial fractures in the elderly. *J. Bone Jt. Surg. Am.* **2009**, *91*, 1868–1873. [CrossRef] [PubMed]
3. Bell, J.E.; Leung, B.C.; Spratt, K.F.; Koval, K.J.; Weinstein, J.D.; Goodman, D.C.; Tosteson, A.N. Trends and variation in incidence, surgical treatment, and repeat surgery of proximal humeral fractures in the elderly. *J. Bone Jt. Surg. Am.* **2011**, *93*, 121–131. [CrossRef] [PubMed]
4. Huttunen, T.T.; Launonen, A.P.; Berg, H.E.; Lepola, V.; Felländer-Tsai, L.; Mattila, V.M. Trends in the incidence of clavicle fractures and surgical repair in Sweden: 2001–2012. *J. Bone Jt. Surg. Am.* **2016**, *98*, 1837–1842. [CrossRef]
5. Miclau, T.; Martin, R.E. The evolution of modern plate osteosynthesis. *Injury* **1997**, *28*, A3–A6. [CrossRef]
6. Hernigou, P.; Pariat, J. History of internal fixation with plates (part 2): New developments after World War II; compressing plates and locked plates. *Int. Orthop.* **2017**, *41*, 1489–1500. [CrossRef]
7. Kingsly, P.; Sathish, M.; Ismail, N.D.M. Comparative analysis of functional outcome of anatomical precontoured locking plate versus reconstruction plate in the management of displaced midshaft clavicular fractures. *J. Orthop. Surg.* **2019**, *27*, 2309499018820351. [CrossRef]
8. Milner, S.A.; Davis, T.R.; Muir, K.R.; Greenwood, D.C.; Doherty, M. Long-term outcome after tibial shaft fracture: Is malunion important? *J. Bone Jt. Surg. Am.* **2002**, *84*, 971–980. [CrossRef]
9. Shin, E.K.; Jupiter, J.B. Current concepts in the management of distal radius fractures. *Acta Chir. Orthop. Traumatol. Cechoslov.* **2007**, *74*, 233–246.
10. Patel, I.; Young, J.; Washington, A.; Vaidya, R. Malunion of the Tibia: A systematic review. *Medicina* **2022**, *58*, 389. [CrossRef]
11. Kwok, C.S.; Crossman, P.T.; Loizou, C.L. Plate versus nail for distal tibial fractures: A systematic review and meta-analysis. *J. Orthop. Trauma* **2014**, *28*, 542–548. [CrossRef] [PubMed]
12. Mao, Z.; Wang, G.; Zhang, L.; Zhang, L.; Chen, S.; Du, H.; Zhao, Y.; Tang, P. Intramedullary nailing versus plating for distal tibia fractures without articular involvement: A meta-analysis. *J. Orthop. Surg. Res.* **2015**, *10*, 95. [CrossRef] [PubMed]
13. Yu, J.; Li, L.; Wang, T.; Sheng, L.; Huo, Y.; Yin, Z.; Gu, G.; He, W. Intramedullary nail versus plate treatments for distal tibial fractures: A meta-analysis. *Int. J. Surg.* **2015**, *16*, 60–68. [CrossRef] [PubMed]

14. Vallier, H.A.; Cureton, B.A.; Patterson, B.M. Randomized, prospective comparison of plate versus intramedullary nail fixation for distal tibia shaft fractures. *J. Orthop. Trauma* **2011**, *25*, 736–741. [CrossRef]
15. Eken, G.; Ermutlu, C.; Durak, K.; Atici, T.; Sarisozen, B.; Cakar, A. Minimally invasive plate osteosynthesis for short oblique diaphyseal tibia fractures: Does fracture site affect the outcomes? *J. Int. Med. Res.* **2020**, *48*, 300060520965402. [CrossRef]
16. Abdi, R.; Aboobakri, M. The use of combined 3.5 LCP unicortical plate and nail fixation in proximal tibia fractures and prevention of valgus and anterior angulation. *J. Surg. Trauma* **2016**, *4*, 7–10.
17. Jeong, H.; Yoo, J.D.; Koh, Y.D.; Sohn, H.S. Omparative Study of Intramedullary Nailing and Plate for Metaphyseal Fractures of the Distal Tibia. *J. Korean Fract. Soc.* **2007**, *20*, 154–160. [CrossRef]
18. Strauss, E.J.; Schwarzkopf, R.; Kummer, F.; Egol, K.A. The current status of locked plating: The good, the bad, and the ugly. *J. Orthop. Trauma* **2008**, *22*, 479–486. [CrossRef]
19. Cronier, P.; Piétu, G.; Dujardin, C.; Bigorre, N.; Ducellier, F.; Gérard, R. The concept of locking plates. *Orthop. Traumatol. Surg. Res.* **2010**, *96*, S17–S36. [CrossRef]
20. Durusoy, S.; Akdoğan, V.; Paksoy, A.E. Do three-dimensional modeling and printing technologies have an impact on the surgical success of percutaneous transsacral screw fixation? *Jt. Dis. Relat. Surg.* **2020**, *31*, 273–280. [CrossRef]
21. Surucu, S.; Aydin, M.; Batma, A.G.; Karasahin, D.; Mahiroğulları, M. Evaluation of the patient satisfaction of using a 3D printed medical casting in fracture treatment. *Jt. Dis. Relat. Surg.* **2022**, *33*, 180–186. [CrossRef] [PubMed]
22. Yang, L.; Shang, X.W.; Fan, J.N.; He, Z.X.; Wang, J.J.; Liu, M.; Zhuang, Y.; Ye, C. Application of 3D printing in the surgical planning of trimalleolar fracture and doctor-patient communication. *Biomed. Res. Int.* **2016**, *2016*, 2482086. [CrossRef] [PubMed]
23. Kang, H.J.; Kim, B.S.; Kim, S.M.; Kim, Y.M.; Kim, H.N.; Park, J.Y.; Cho, J.H.; Choi, Y. Can preoperative 3D printing change surgeon's operative plan for distal tibia fracture? *Biomed. Res. Int.* **2019**, *2019*, 7059413. [CrossRef] [PubMed]
24. Yammine, K.; Karbala, J.; Maalouf, A.; Daher, J.; Assi, C. Clinical outcomes of the use of 3D printing models in fracture management: A meta-analysis of randomized studies. *Eur. J. Trauma Emerg. Surg.* **2021**, *12*, 1–13. [CrossRef] [PubMed]
25. Xiong, L.; Li, X.; Li, H.; Chen, Z.; Xiao, T. The efficacy of 3D printing-assisted surgery for traumatic fracture: A meta-analysis. *Postgrad. Med. J.* **2019**, *95*, 414–419. [CrossRef]
26. Zhang, W.; Ji, Y.; Wang, X.; Liu, J.; Li, D. Can the recovery of lower limb fractures be achieved by use of 3D printing mirror model? *Injury* **2017**, *48*, 2485–2495. [CrossRef]
27. Jeong, H.S.; Park, K.J.; Kil, K.M.; Chong, S.; Eun, H.J.; Lee, T.S.; Lee, J.P. Minimally invasive plate osteosynthesis using 3D printing for shaft fractures of clavicles: Technical note. *Arch. Orthop. Trauma Surg.* **2014**, *134*, 1551–1555. [CrossRef] [PubMed]
28. Upex, P.; Jouffroy, P.; Riouallon, G. Application of 3D printing for treating fractures of both columns of the acetabulum: Benefit of pre-contouring plates on the mirrored healthy pelvis. *Orthop. Traumatol. Surg. Res.* **2017**, *103*, 331–334. [CrossRef]
29. Wang, C.; Chen, Y.; Wang, L.; Wang, D.; Gu, C.; Lin, X.; Liu, H.; Chen, J.; Wen, X.; Liu, Y.; et al. Three-dimensional printing of patient-specific plates for the treatment of acetabular fractures involving quadrilateral plate disruption. *BMC Musculoskelet. Disord.* **2020**, *21*, 451. [CrossRef]
30. Zhang, D.; Qiu, D.; Gibson, M.A.; Zheng, Y.; Fraser, H.L.; StJohn, D.H.; Easton, M.A. Additive manufacturing of ultrafine-grained high-strength titanium alloys. *Nature* **2019**, *576*, 91–95. [CrossRef]
31. Barriobero-Vila, P.; Gussone, J.; Stark, A.; Schell, N.; Haubrich, J.; Requena, G. Peritectic titanium alloys for 3D printing. *Nat. Commun.* **2018**, *9*, 3426. [CrossRef] [PubMed]

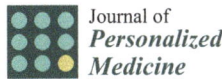

Article

Three-Dimensional Evaluation of Isodose Radiation Volumes in Cases of Severe Mandibular Osteoradionecrosis for the Prediction of Recurrence after Segmental Resection

Haye H. Glas [1,*], Joep Kraeima [1], Silke Tribius [2], Frank K. J. Leusink [3], Carsten Rendenbach [4], Max Heiland [4], Carmen Stromberger [5], Ashkan Rashad [6], Clifton D. Fuller [7], Abdallah S. R. Mohamed [7], Stephen Y. Lai [7,8] and Max J. H. Witjes [1]

[1] Department of Oral and Maxillofacial Surgery, University Medical Center Groningen, University of Groningen, 9713GZ Groningen, The Netherlands; j.kraeima@umcg.nl (J.K.); m.j.h.witjes@umcg.nl (M.J.H.W.)
[2] Hermann-Holthusen-Institute for Radiation Oncolo Gy, Asklepios Hospital St. Georg, University Medical Center Hamburg-Eppendorf, 20246 Hamburg, Germany; s.tribius@asklepios.com
[3] Department of Oral and Maxillofacial Surgery, Amsterdam University Medical Center, 1100DD Amsterdam, The Netherlands; f.leusink@amsterdamumc.nl
[4] Department of Oral and Maxillofacial Surgery, Charité–Universitätsmedizin, Corporate Member of Freie Universität Berlin, Humboldt-Universität zu Berlin and Berlin Institute of Health, 12203 Berlin, Germany; carsten.rendenbach@charite.de (C.R.); max.heiland@charite.de (M.H.)
[5] Department of Radiation Oncolo Gy and Radiation Therapy, Charité–Universitätsmedizin, Corporate Member of Freie Universität Berlin, Humboldt-Universität zu Berlin and Berlin Institute of Health, 12203 Berlin, Germany; carmen.stromberger@charite.de
[6] Department of Oral, Maxillofacial and Facial Plastic Surgery, RWTH Aachen University Hospital, 52074 Aachen, Germany; arashad@ukaachen.de
[7] Department of Radiation Oncolo Gy, Division of Radiation Oncolo Gy, The University of Texas MD Anderson Cancer Center, Houston, TX 77030, USA; cdfuller@mdanderson.org (C.D.F.); asmohamed@mdanderson.org (A.S.R.M.); sylai@mdanderson.org (S.Y.L.)
[8] Department of Head and Neck Surgery, Division of Surgery, The University of Texas MD Anderson Cancer Center, Houston, TX 77030, USA
* Correspondence: mka@umcg.nl; Tel.: +31-(0)50-361-25-61

Citation: Glas, H.H.; Kraeima, J.; Tribius, S.; Leusink, F.K.J.; Rendenbach, C.; Heiland, M.; Stromberger, C.; Rashad, A.; Fuller, C.D.; Mohamed, A.S.R.; et al. Three-Dimensional Evaluation of Isodose Radiation Volumes in Cases of Severe Mandibular Osteoradionecrosis for the Prediction of Recurrence after Segmental Resection. *J. Pers. Med.* **2022**, *12*, 834. https://doi.org/10.3390/jpm12050834

Academic Editor: David Alan Rizzieri

Received: 13 April 2022
Accepted: 16 May 2022
Published: 20 May 2022

Publisher's Note: MDPI stays neutral with regard to jurisdictional claims in published maps and institutional affiliations.

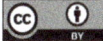

Copyright: © 2022 by the authors. Licensee MDPI, Basel, Switzerland. This article is an open access article distributed under the terms and conditions of the Creative Commons Attribution (CC BY) license (https://creativecommons.org/licenses/by/4.0/).

Abstract: Background: Pre-operative margin planning for the segmental resection of affected bone in mandibular osteoradionecrosis (ORN) is difficult. The aim of this study was to identify a possible relation between the received RT dose, exposed bone volume and the progression of ORN after segmental mandibular resection. Method: Patients diagnosed with grade 3-4 ORN for which a segmental resection was performed were included in the study. Three-dimensional reconstructions of RT isodose volumes were fused with postoperative imaging. The primary outcome was the recurrence of ORN after segmental resection. Subsequently, RT exposed mandibular bone volumes were calculated and the location of the bone cuts relative to the isodose volumes were assessed. Results: Five out of thirty-three patients developed recurrent ORN after segmental mandibular resection. All cases with recurrent ORN were resected inside an isodose volume of $\geq$56 Gy. The absolute mandibular volume radiated with 56 Gy was significantly smaller in the recurrent group (10.9 mL vs. 30.7 mL, $p = 0.006$), as was the proportion of the mandible radiated with 56 Gy (23% vs. 45%, $p = 0.013$). Conclusion: The volume of radiated bone was not predictive for risk of progression. The finding that recurrent ORN occurred with bone resection margins within the 56 Gy isodose volume suggests that this could serve as a starting point for the pre-operative planning of reducing the risk of ORN recurrence.

Keywords: osteoradionecrosis; mandible; radiotherapy; surgery; computer assisted surgery; virtual surgical planning

1. Introduction

Osteoradionecrosis (ORN) of the mandible is a late complication of radiotherapy (RT). ORN most commonly occurs in the tooth-bearing body of the mandible [1]. It is described as exposed irradiated bone that fails to heal over a period of three months without evidence of a persisting or recurrent tumour [2]. Incidence of ORN is reported to occur in 1–15% of head and neck cancer patients with a median latency of 1 to 2 years after RT [1,3–7]. Factors such as the received RT-dose, the volume of mandible included in the planning target volume (PTV) as well as the fractionation schedule are known to influence the occurrence of ORN [3,4,6,8,9]. Other risk factors associated with the development of ORN are surgery to the mandible, dental condition and pre- or post-RT tooth extractions, as well as continued smoking [1,5,10–13]. There is no association between concomitant chemotherapy and the incidence of ORN [12]. The initiation of ORN is mainly reported after traumatic events to the bone but is also known to occur spontaneously [14,15].

Mental neuropathy, dehiscent bone or fistulas may be predictors for ORN as well as medication-related osteonecrosis of the jaw (MRONJ); however, ORN patients demonstrate significantly more pathological fractures, skin fistulae and pain compared to MRONJ [16,17]. Despite some similarities, ORN and MRONJ are considered two distinct pathological entities [16].

The treatment of patients with ORN depends on the extent of the affected bone and may consist of antibiotics, debridement, sequestrectomy, hyperbaric oxygen therapy, or a combination of the aforementioned techniques [18]. Treatment of severe mandibular ORN often requires the surgical removal of the affected bone and segmental resection is often necessary. ORN of the jaw is often classified into several stages that describe the severity or progression of the disease. The classification used by Marx et al. defines three stages of ORN, in which the third stage includes pathological fractures, orocutaneous fistulas or radiographic evidence of resorption of the inferior border.

The risk of developing ORN is associated with a dose of >60 Gy to the bone [8,19,20], or a mean dose to the total mandibular volume of >48 Gy [21]. Additionally, a gross tumour volume (GTV) dose of >54 Gy is related to an increased risk of developing ORN [4]. Furthermore, the risk of developing ORN is also reported to be related to the volume of bone and the received RT dose. Emami et al. reported a 5% risk of developing ORN within the 5 years following RT when 2/3 of the mandible is radiated with more than 60 Gy, which is equal to more than 65 Gy when approximately 1/3 of the mandible is exposed [9]. Tsai et al. reported a matched case–control analysis, with a significant difference between the volume of the mandible in the two groups receiving doses between 50 Gy (V_{50}) and 60 Gy (V_{60}) [6]. Abdallah et al. reported on a case–control matched study with significant higher dose-volume histogram () bins from V35 to v73 in the ORN cohort [21]. A DVH is used to relate radiation dose to tissue volume. It can be concluded that the risk of ORN increases with radiation dose and radiated mandibular volume, with an incremental increasing risk for ORN at doses of above 50 Gy.

Currently, the position of bone cuts for mandibular segmental resection are based on the clinical inspection of the lesion and pre-operative imaging such as panoramic X-rays or (CB)CT/MRI. The use of Technetium-bone scans has been described as a method to identify the affected bone [22]. Using DCE-MRI, differences in vascular leakiness can be measured between affected and healthy bone tissue [23]. However, surgeons often struggle with the decision of where to make cuts in the mandible and the resulting margins. The most commonly used technique is to remove bone until healthy, bleeding bone is visible [24]. Others have described using tetracycline as a fluorescent marker to discriminate between vital and necrotic bone [25–27]. As was described by Kraeima et al., the 3D- visualization of the isodose lines obtained using RT planned with IMRT in relation to the mandibular bone can support preoperative planning [28]. This method provides a potential decision-making tool that can be used pre-operatively. However, sufficient data on the relationship between the received RT dose and the ideal location for the bone cuts when a segmental mandibular resection is performed are not available. Defining this relationship is important in order to determine a cut-off dose that may possibly be used for the pre-operative planning of the surgical resection or placement of screws for fixating osteosynthesis materials.

This study describes a retrospective analysis of an international multi-institutional database for patients with severe ORN that required surgical treatment. The aim of the study was to identify the relationship between the received RT dose, exposed bone volume and progression of ORN after segmental mandibular resection in order to support the preoperative planning of the bone cuts.

2. Materials and Method

2.1. Patients

An international consortium of medical centres collected retrospective data on patients who underwent segmental mandibular resection as treatment for ORN. The selection focused on patients who developed severe (Marx classification grade 3) ORN after RT/chemoRT and were treated in the following centres: University of Texas MD Anderson Cancer Center (Houston, TX, USA), Charité-Universitätsmedizin Berlin (Berlin, Germany), University Medical Center Hamburg-Eppendorf (Hamburg, Germany), Amsterdam University Medical Center (Amsterdam, the Netherlands) and the University Medical Center Groningen (Groningen, the Netherlands). Written informed consent was obtained from all subjects involved in the study. The study was approved by the ethical committee (Berlin EA1/206/18).

Inclusion criteria were as follows: (1) Patients diagnosed with Marx grade 3 ORN of the mandible after IMRT for which a segmental resection was performed; (2) patients who underwent IMRT with curative intent as part of their initial treatment after the confirmed pathological diagnosis of oral or oropharyngeal squamous cell carcinoma; (3) availability of the following data: radiotherapy-CT scan and radiation plan (DICOM-RT) to reconstruct 3D-isodose fields and the postoperative imaging data to derive the performed resection, either by CT scan or orthopantomogram (OPT). Furthermore, patients who received brachytherapy or previous head and neck RT were excluded.

The following patient characteristics were recorded: age, gender, smoking and alcohol consumption, tumour stage and location, primary treatment (surgery, RT, chemoradiation or a combination of aforementioned), months between RT and diagnosis of ORN, dental status, HBO therapy, RT dose and fractionation schedule. The dental status was retrieved from clinical files, including performed extractions or the invasive treatment of any other conditions. If such data were not available, patients were marked edentulous when the RT planning CT did not reveal any elements.

2.2. Processing of Imaging Data

For every case, the RT planning CT scan was selected for the 3D-segmentation of the bone (e.g., the mandible). The DICOM-RT clinical treatment plans were uploaded to the RT planning software research database (Mirada, Mirada Medical, Oxford, UK) and fused with the selected CT dataset. The 56 Gy and PTV isodose curves were visualized and exported as RTSS files. Subsequently, these RTSS files were fused with the RT planning CT using a similar conversion method to that described by Kraeima et al. [29], using Matlab 2018a (MathWorks, Natick, MA, USA). After data fusion, a 3D-virtual model of both the involved bone, 56 Gy and PTV isodose volumes were produced using ProPlan CMF 3.0 (Materialise, Leuven, Belgium). Figure 1 presents a stepwise overview of the workflow.

Postoperative imaging was used to derive the margins of the performed segmental resection, using either a CT scan or OPT. When a postoperative CT scan was available, 3D-segmentation of the resected mandible was performed and registered with the 3D RT reconstruction. When the shape of the mandible significantly changed due to the reconstruction, this registration was performed twice, once for each segment. Hereafter, cutting planes superimposing the performed resection onto the RT bone model were constructed. In case an OPT was used, resection planes were translated manually using screen-to-screen comparison onto the RT bone model.

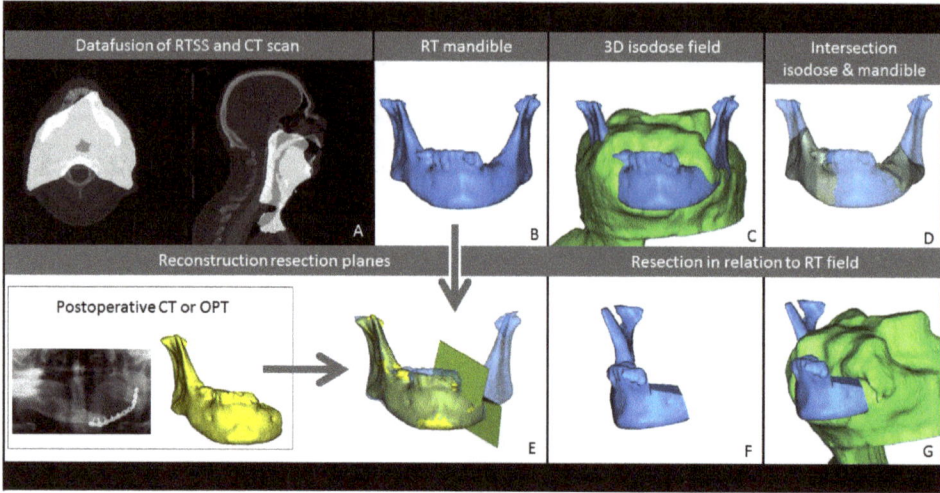

Figure 1. Describing the workflow of data fusion and segmentation, including reconstruction of the performed segmental resection. (**A**). Data fusion of radiotherapy planning files (RTSS) and RT CT scan. (**B**). 3D model of the mandible from RT CT scan. (**C**). In green, the 3D reconstruction of the 56 Gy isodose volume. (**D**). In yellow, the volume of the mandible radiated with 56 Gy (Vm56). (**E**). Reconstruction of performed segmental resection using either a postoperative CT or OPT. (**F**). Mandible after segmental resection. (**G**). Mandible after segmental resection in relation to the 56 Gy isodose volume (V56).

2.3. Measurements

Volume measurements were performed on the combined dataset, including total mandible volume (Vm), 56 Gy and PTV isodose volumes (V56, V-PTV), volume of mandible inside the 56 Gy (Vm56) and PTV (Vm-PTV) isodose volume. The PTV resembled the high-dose volume and included the gross tumour volume (GTV) and the clinical target volume with an additional set-up margin. The PTV dose is typically equal or higher than 56 Gy. Further measurements included volume of the resection of the mandible (VmR), and residual volume of V56 and V-PTV after resection surgery (Vm56R, Vm-PTV-R). Besides absolute volumes, the distribution of the volumes was calculated as a percentage of total mandibular volume. Furthermore, for each resection, we assessed whether the resection was performed inside the Vm56 and Vm-PTV volume. If the resection was performed inside the Vm56 volume, the involvement of the lingual and/or buccal cortex was noted. Figure 2 illustrates an example of lingual involvement in the osteotomy with the Vm56. Moreover, the progression of ORN after segmental resection was used as an outcome measure. A Kolmogorov–Smirnov analysis for normal distribution was performed. A student's *t*-test for normally distributed data and the Mann–Whitney U (MWW) test for skewed data were used to detect significant differences between recurrent and non-recurrent cases.

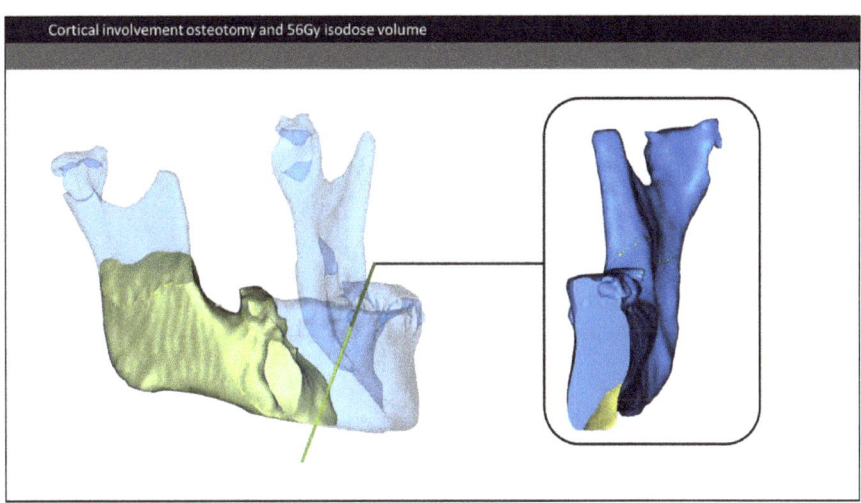

Figure 2. Cortical involvement osteotomy and 56 Gy isodose volume. On the left, an overview of the mandible and the 56 Gy isodose volume (yellow). The osteotomy plane is visualized in green. On the right side, a view perpendicular to the osteotomy plane. In this case, only the lingual cortex is involved.

3. Results

3.1. Patient Characteristics

A total of 33 patients who underwent segmental mandibulectomy for severe ORN following RT/chemoRT were included in the study. Patients were treated for primary ORN between 2008 and 2018. Follow-up after initial ORN surgery was 69 months (range 19–142 months). Five patients were diagnosed with recurrence of ORN after initial segmental resection. A complete list of all patient characteristics can be found in Table 1.

Table 1. Patient characteristics.

			Value	%
Age				
		Median (range)	60	(43–76)
sex				
		male	21	64%
		Female	12	36%
Smoking status				
		Never	6	23%
		Former	11	42%
		Current	9	35%
		unknown	7	
Smoking pack-year				
		Mean (SD)	31	(23)
Alcohol history				
		occasional	5	19%
		Former	11	41%

Table 1. *Cont.*

		Value	%
	Current	13	48%
	unknown	6	
Tumour location			
	Base of tonque	11	48%
	Tonsil	8	35%
	Other	4	17%
	unknown	10	
T stage			
	T1	1	3%
	T2	12	38%
	T3	6	19%
	T4	13	41%
	unknown	1	
N stage			
	N0	6	19%
	N1	5	16%
	N2	21	66%
	unknown	1	
Primary treatment			
	RT	3	9%
	Surgery + RT	7	21%
	RCT	20	61%
	Surgery + RCT	3	9%
Time RT-ORN			
	Months (range)	28	(1–76)
Reconstruction method			
	Fibula (unknown)	12	
		21	(21)
Follow-up initial ORN			
	Months (range)	69	(19–142)
Dental status			
	Edentulous	11	33%
	dental extractions	16	59%
	unknown	6	
HBO therapy		18	55%
Radiation dose			
	Median (range)	70 Gy	(56–72)
Radiation fractions			
	Median (range)	33	(28–45)
	RT = radiotherapy		
	RCT = radiotherapy + chemotherapy		

A total of 75 patients diagnosed with severe ORN were assessed. Forty-two patients were excluded from the analysis. Reasons for exclusion included no segmental resection (12), incomplete RT planning data or unavailable data for reconstruction (13), incomplete postoperative imaging data (11), prior RT (3), additional brachytherapy (1), total radiation dose <56 Gy (1) and unavailable patient record (1).

3.2. Recurrent Cases

A total of five patients were diagnosed with recurrent ORN after mandibular segmental resection, with initial diagnoses of ORN occurring 16.2 months (range 1–34) after RT. The median age of patients was 60 years (range 53–66 years). The mean radiation dose was 64 Gy (SD 6.4 Gy). Figure 3 illustrates the recurrent ORN cases, including the radiated mandibular volume, performed resection and location of the recurrent ORN. Four patients were edentulous at the time of RT and three patients presented osteosynthesis material in situ during RT.

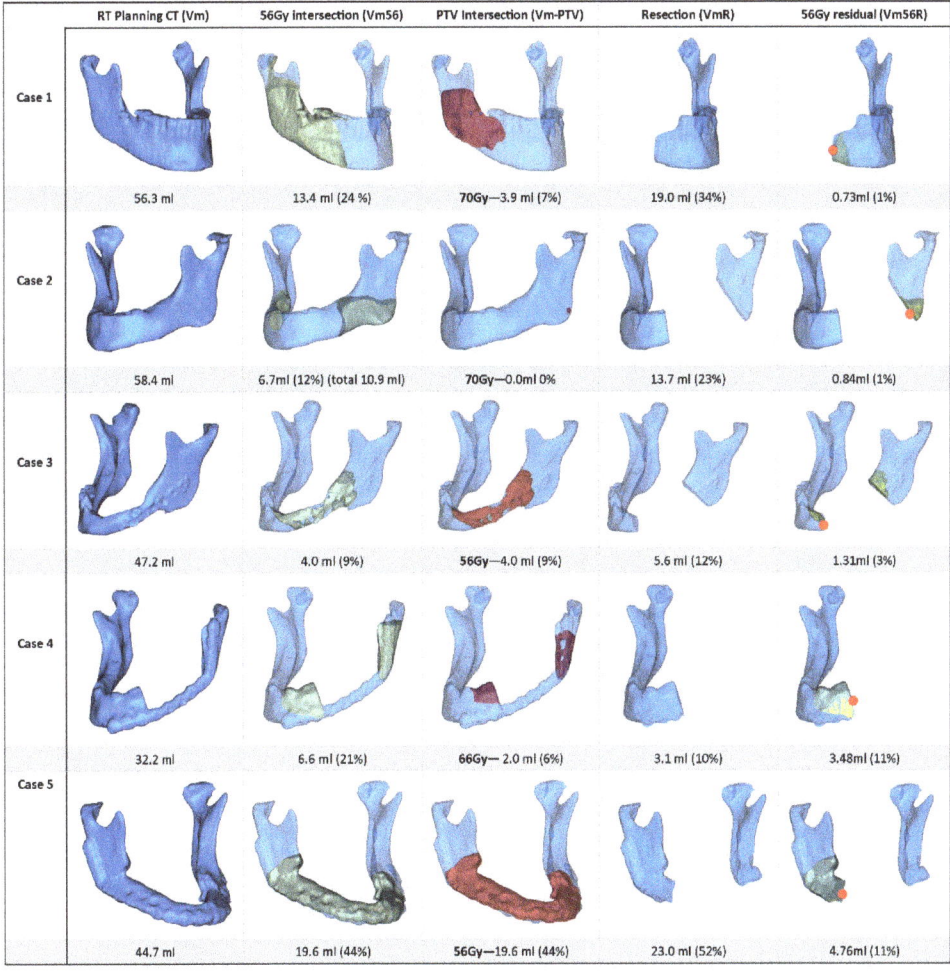

Figure 3. Overview of patients with recurrence of ORN after segmental resection. The first column illustrates the 3D segmentation of the mandible during radiotherapy, representing the total

mandibular volume (Vm). The second column illustrates, in yellow, the volume of the mandible inside the 56 Gy isodose (Vm56). The third column, in red, represents the volume of the mandible inside the PTV (Vm-PTV). The forth column shows the postoperative situation after segmental resection (VmR). The last column shows the residual volume of Vm56 after resection surgery (Vm56R). The red dots in the last column indicate the location of the ORN recurrence.

3.3. Measurements

The mean mandible volume was 62.7 mL (range 26.4–95mL). On average, 42% (range 9–83%) of the mandible was radiated with at least 56 Gy (Vm56/Vm), and 15% (range 0–51%) of the mandible received the PTV dose, which ranged from 56 Gy to 72 Gy. On average 35% (range 7–78%) of the mandible was resected. The total mandibular volume of the recurrent ORN group was smaller compared to the non-recurrent group (65.4 mL vs. 47.8 mL, t-test $p = 0.045$). Additionally, Vm56 volume was significantly smaller in the recurrent group (10.9 mL vs. 30.7ml, t-test $p = 0.006$). The proportion of mandible radiated with 56 Gy was smaller for the recurrent group than for the non-recurrent group (23% vs. 45% (MWW $p = 0.013$)). Resections performed in the non-recurrent group included a larger proportion (37%) of the total mandibular volume compared to the recurrent group (26%), although this was not significant (MWW $p = 0.268$). Two recurrences of ORN in patients occurred for those who received the highest doses of RT of 70 Gy or more while 20 patients showed no recurrences. The overall volume measures were smaller in recurrent cases than in non-recurrent cases. A complete overview of the volume measurements and volume distribution is provided in Table 2.

Table 2. Mean, minimum and maximum volumes of mandible and RT isodose fields. Volume of mandible (Vm), 56 Gy and PTV isodose volume (V56, V-PTV). Volume mandible inside 56 Gy isodose and PTV (Vm56, Vm-PTV). Volume of resection (VmR) and residual volume of Vm56 and Vm-PTV after resection (Vm56R, Vm-PTV-R). Significant differences between recurrent and non-recurrent group are highlighted in red.

		Vm	V56	V-PTV	Vm56	Vm-PTV	Vm56R	Vm-PTV-R	VmR	Vm56/Vm	Vm-PTV/Vm	VmR/Vm
Total (n = 33)	Mean (mL)	62.7	772.8	221.5	27.7	9.2	9.6	3.3	39.4	42%	15%	35%
	min	26.4	33.8	0.0	4.0	0.0	0.0	0.0	23.9	9%	0%	7%
	max	95.0	1760.9	623.2	77.5	38.6	53.1	31.4	36.0	83%	51%	78%
Non-recurrent (n = 28)	Mean (mL)	65.4	843.5	238.6	30.7	9.8	10.9	3.8	40.3	45%	15%	37%
	min	26.4	183.6	0.0	4.5	0.0	0.0	0.0	23.9	10%	0%	7%
	max	95.0	1760.9	623.2	77.5	38.6	53.1	31.4	36.0	83%	51%	78%
Recurrent (n = 5)	Mean (mL)	47.8	376.9	125.7	10.9	5.9	2.2	0.0	34.8	23%	13%	26%
	min	32.2	33.8	33.8	4.0	0.0	0.7	0.0	29.1	9%	0%	10%
	max	58.4	763.0	212.1	19.6	19.6	4.8	0.0	35.1	44%	44%	52%
>70 Gy Non-recurrent (n = 20)	Mean (mL)	67.8	950.7	235.6	29.9	6.7	7.7	1.5	43.7	43%	10%	34%
	min	26.4	183.6	0.0	6.7	0.0	0.0	0.0	23.9	12%	0%	7%
	max	95.0	1760.9	604.8	77.5	33.7	32.5	10.2	42.2	83%	44%	63%
>70 Gy Recurrent (n = 2)	Mean (mL)	57.3	751.3	196.7	12.2	1.9	0.8	0.0	41.0	21%	3%	29%
	min	56.3	739.7	181.3	10.9	0.0	0.7	0.0	42.6	19%	0%	23%
	max	58.4	763.0	212.1	13.4	3.9	0.8	0.0	39.4	24%	7%	34%

A total of 60 osteotomy planes were reconstructed (8 recurrent cases, 52 non-recurrent cases). In total, 14 resections were outside the Vm56. Thus, the margin was in bone that received a lower RT dose. Of the 46 resections inside the Vm56, 10 planes intersected the Vm56 at the lingual cortex only. The remaining 36 resections intersected the Vm56 in both the lingual and buccal cortex. Of the eight osteotomies in the recurrent ORN group, five intersected the Vm56 bicortically, one on the lingual side and the remaining two were performed outside the Vm56, thus in bone with a dose of less than 56 Gy.

4. Discussion

In the present study, five out of thirty-three patients developed a recurrence of ORN after segmental resection. Two of the five patients received a maximum RT dose of 56 Gy and for the other three patients the ORN recurred in a mandibular volume that was exposed to more than 56 Gy RT. No recurrence was observed with margins placed in the mandibular volume exposed to less than 56 Gy. Although not significantly different, the resection volumes in the non-recurrent ORN group were larger than in the recurrent ORN group, possibly indicating that sufficiently large resection volumes of radiated bone may reduce the chance of recurrence. This study is a first attempt to involve radiation dose in surgical decision making in the treatment of ORN. Because of the retrospective nature of the study, the data were focused on what could be reliably extracted, the placement of the bone cut, the isodose and the progression of ORN.

Aiming to place the bone margin outside the 56 Gy volume may reduce the risk of ORN recurrence. Although this concept is supported by general findings in the literature that the risk of ORN increases incrementally with doses of more than 50 Gy, the data from the current cohort do not support this [4,6,8,19,21]. Moreover, it has been suggested that the risk of recurrent ORN after surgical resection is associated with multiple factors and should most likely be considered as such [1,3–11,13]. Thus, the approach of making resection-margin decisions based on isodose distribution needs to be approached with caution. From this data, the concept of always placing the bone margins outside the 56 Gy isodose volume could not be applied uniformly.

Studer at al. reported about 42 patients for whom a mean mandible volume of 4.6% received the prescribed dose (71 Gy) [7]. Compared to our cohort of patients who received a prescribed dose of a minimum of 70 Gy, we found 10% for the non-recurrent ORN group and 3% for the recurrent ORN group. According to Emami et al., the risk of developing an ORN is 5% in 5 years if one third of the mandible is exposed to 65 Gy, or if two thirds is exposed to 60 Gy [9]. In our study, on average, 42% of the mandible received a dose of 56 Gy. However, for the recurrent cases this proportion was lower (23%) than for the non-recurrent ORN cases (45%). This is also lower than the DVH constraints of V58 < 25% proposed by Abdallah et al. [21].

Mandibular surgery increases the risk of the development of ORN [4], where marginal or periosteal bone resection impose the highest risk, followed by segmental or no resection [19]. In the recurrent ORN group, three of the five patients had osteosynthesis material in place during RT/chemoRT. In two of these patients, a segmental resection and reconstruction was performed during primary resection. One patient underwent reconstruction with a fibula graft, the other solely with osteosynthesis. The third case had a mandibular fracture that was sustained during radical surgery, for which internal fixation was indicated. In the non-recurrent ORN group, only four of the twenty-eight patients had already undergone reconstructive surgery. This might also explain the difference in the total mandibular bone volume at the time of RT between the recurrent and non-recurrent ORN group. The resection in recurrent case 4 consisted of removing the condyle and osteosyntheses material, and there was no bone cutting. However, this case is considered as a bicortical involvement of the osteotomy at the Vm56 volume, because the Vm56 was not completely removed during surgery. For recurrent case 5, one of the osteotomies was performed in the fibula graft and not in the mandibular bone. For the same reason mentioned before, this osteotomy was also considered as bicortical involvement.

In this study, a non-systematic analysis of retrospective data on ORN patients was conducted to establish evidence to support potential dose–volume criteria for pre-operative decision making for 3D-virtual surgical planning. Data from 33 patients were used from an initial cohort of 75 patients (incomplete records in 42 cases), emphasizing the need for a multicentre approach. Despite the multicentre approach, only a limited number of patients could be included. The limited data availability and the resulting statistical power is the main limitation of this study. Moreover, as treatment and surgical reconstruction techniques differ between patients, but also between surgeons and health centres, comparing individual patients is even more challenging. In addition, ORN is a multifactorial disorder, and due to the retrospective nature of the study, not all factors could be included. We did not find a relation between the proportion of recurrences and the RT dose or dose-volumes. Perhaps the group was too small to draw conclusions related to RT dose and dose volumes. This study was not set up as an investigation of the causes of ORN, but for the risk of recurrence. Therefore, the data retrieved from these cases should not be viewed similarly to those in previous reports on the relationship of RT dose, dose volumes and the risk of developing ORN. The unexpected finding that mandibular RT dose volumes were smaller in the recurrent ORN group is perhaps more a consequence of all patients already having ORN and less related to recurrence.

The surgical technique and choices regarding the placement of the bone cuts and reconstruction are relevant for the risk of the progression of ORN. The risk of ORN progression is not solely based on the RT dose given to the bone. Other factors related to surgery, such as vascularization of the remaining bone, quality of the covering soft tissue as well as patient-related factors, including smoking and health status. Placing the bone margin in the isodose volume with the lowest risk of the recurrence of ORN may be just one factor in the process. The importance of planning the bone margin is even more essential for 3D-surgical planning of the bone reconstruction. The traditional surgical approach would be free-hand resection and shaping of the composite flap in the OR without 3D-virtual planning. In the OR, regardless of the decision to utilize 3D-planning, the surgeon is faced with the problem of where to cut and the following question remains: 'is bleeding bone a safe criterion?'.

5. Conclusions

All of the patients who experienced the progression of ORN after the surgical removal of the affected mandibular bone were resected inside the 56 Gy volume. Although the volume measurements alone are not predictive for progression, the authors suggest that the use of 3D-isodose volumes may be an option to avoid areas at risk for ORN during one-stage resection and reconstructive surgery. This approach warrants further evaluation.

Author Contributions: Conceptualization, H.H.G., J.K. and M.J.H.W.; methodolo Gy, H.H.G., J.K., S.T., F.K.J.L., C.R., M.H., C.S., A.R., C.D.F., A.S.R.M., S.Y.L. and M.J.H.W.; software, H.H.G. and J.K.; validation, H.H.G., J.K. and M.J.H.W.; investigation, H.H.G., J.K., S.T., F.K.J.L., C.R., M.H., C.S., A.R., C.D.F., A.S.R.M., S.Y.L. and M.J.H.W.; resources, H.H.G., J.K., S.T., F.K.J.L., C.R., M.H., C.S., A.R., C.D.F., A.S.R.M., S.Y.L. and M.J.H.W.; data curation, H.H.G.; writing—original draft preparation, H.H.G.; writing—review and editing, H.H.G., J.K., S.T., F.K.J.L., C.R., M.H., C.S., A.R., C.D.F., A.S.R.M., S.Y.L. and M.J.H.W.; visualization, H.H.G.; supervision, J.K. and M.J.H.W.; project administration, H.H.G., J.K. and M.J.H.W.; funding acquisition, not applicable. All authors have read and agreed to the published version of the manuscript.

Funding: This research received no external funding.

Institutional Review Board Statement: The work was conducted in accordance with the Declaration of Helsinki. The study was approved by ethical committee: Berlin EA1/206/18.

Informed Consent Statement: Written informed consent was obtained from all subjects involved in the study.

Data Availability Statement: The data that support the findings of this study are available from the corresponding author, H.H.G, upon reasonable request.

Conflicts of Interest: The authors declare no conflict of interest.

Abbreviations

3D	Three-dimensional
GTV	Gross tumour volume
DVH	Dose volume histogram
IMRT	Intensity modulated radiotherapy
MRONJ	Medication-related osteonecrosis of the jaw
ORN	Osteoradionecrosis
PTV	Planning target volume
RT	Radiotherapy
Vm	Mandible volume
VSP	Virtual surgical planning

References

1. Reuther, T.; Schuster, T.; Mende, U.; Kübler, A. Osteoradionecrosis of the jaws as a side effect of radiotherapy of head and neck tumour patients—A report of a thirty year retrospective review. *Int. J. Oral Maxillofac. Surg.* **2003**, *32*, 289–295. [CrossRef] [PubMed]
2. Mallya, S.M.; Tetradis, S. Imaging of Radiation- and Medication-Related Osteonecrosis. *Radiol. Clin. N. Am.* **2018**, *56*, 77–89. [CrossRef] [PubMed]
3. Mendenhall, W.M.; Suárez, C.; Genden, E.M.; De Bree, R.; Strojan, P.; Langendijk, J.A.; Mäkitie, A.A.; Smee, R.; Eisbruch, A.; Lee, A.W.; et al. Parameters Associated With Mandibular Osteoradionecrosis. *Am. J. Clin. Oncol. Cancer Clin. Trials* **2018**, *41*, 1276–1280. [CrossRef] [PubMed]
4. Lee, I.J.; Koom, W.S.; Lee, C.G.; Kim, Y.B.; Yoo, S.W.; Keum, K.C.; Kim, G.E.; Choi, E.C.; Cha, I. Risk Factors and Dose–Effect Relationship for Mandibular Osteoradionecrosis in Oral and Oropharyngeal Cancer Patients. *Int. J. Radiat. Oncol. Biol. Phys.* **2009**, *75*, 1084–1091. [CrossRef] [PubMed]
5. Pereira, I.; Firmino, R.; Meira, H.; Vasconcelos, B.; Noronha, V.; Santos, V. Osteoradionecrosis prevalence and associated factors: A ten years retrospective study. *Med. Oral Patol. Oral y Cir. Bucal* **2018**, *23*, e633–e638. [CrossRef] [PubMed]
6. Tsai, C.J.; Hofstede, T.M.; Sturgis, E.M.; Garden, A.S.; Lindberg, M.E.; Wei, Q.; Tucker, S.L.; Dong, L. Osteoradionecrosis and Radiation Dose to the Mandible in Patients With Oropharyngeal Cancer. *Int. J. Radiat. Oncol. Biol. Phys.* **2012**, *85*, 415–420. [CrossRef] [PubMed]
7. Studer, G.; Studer, S.P.; Zwahlen, R.A.; Huguenin, P.; Grätz, K.W.; Lütolf, U.M.; Glanzmann, C. Osteoradionecrosis of the mandible: Minimized risk profile following intensity-modulated radiation therapy (IMRT). *Strahlenther. Onkol.* **2006**, *182*, 283–288. [CrossRef]
8. Murray, C.G.; Herson, J.; Daly, T.E.; Zimmerman, S. Radiation necrosis of the mandible: A 10 year study. Part I. Factors influencing the onset of necrosis. *Int. J. Radiat. Oncol. Biol. Phys.* **1980**, *6*, 543–548. [CrossRef]
9. Emami, B. Tolerance of Normal Tissue to Irradiation. *Int. J. Radiat. Oncol. Biol. Phys.* **1991**, *21*, 109–122. [CrossRef]
10. Aarup-Kristensen, S.; Hansen, C.R.; Forner, L.; Brink, C.; Eriksen, J.G.; Johansen, J. Osteoradionecrosis of the mandible after radiotherapy for head and neck cancer: Risk factors and dose-volume correlations. *Acta Oncol.* **2019**, *58*, 1373–1377. [CrossRef]
11. Manzano, B.R.; Santaella, N.G.; Oliveira, M.A.; Rubira, C.M.F.; de Santos, P.S. Retrospective study of osteoradi-onecrosis in the jaws of patients with head and neck cancer. *J. Korean Assoc. Oral Maxillofac. Surg.* **2019**, *45*, 21–28. [CrossRef] [PubMed]
12. Studer, G.; Grätz, K.W.; Glanzmann, C. Osteoradionecrosis of the Mandibula in Patients Treated with Different Fractionations. *Strahlenther. Onkol.* **2004**, *180*, 233–240. [CrossRef] [PubMed]
13. Glanzmann, C.; Grätz, K. Radionecrosis of the mandibula: A retrospective analysis of the incidence and risk factors. *Radiother. Oncol.* **1995**, *36*, 94–100. [CrossRef]
14. Marx, R.E. A New Concept of Its Pathophysiolo Gy. *Growth* **1983**, *41*, 283–288.
15. Wanifuchi, S.; Akashi, M.; Ejima, Y.; Shinomiya, H.; Minamikawa, T.; Furudoi, S.; Otsuki, N.; Sasaki, R.; Nibu, K.-I.; Komori, T. Cause and occurrence timing of osteoradionecrosis of the jaw: A retrospective study focusing on prophylactic tooth extraction. *Oral Maxillofac. Surg.* **2016**, *20*, 337–342. [CrossRef] [PubMed]
16. Grisar, K.; Schol, M.; Schoenaers, J.; Dormaar, T.; Coropciuc, R.; Poorten, V.V.; Politis, C. Osteoradionecrosis and medication-related osteonecrosis of the jaw: Similarities and differences. *Int. J. Oral Maxillofac. Surg.* **2016**, *45*, 1592–1599. [CrossRef]
17. Fortunato, L.; Amato, M.; Simeone, M.; Bennardo, F.; Barone, S.; Giudice, A. Numb chin syndrome: A reflection of malignancy or a harbinger of MRONJ? A multicenter experience. *J. Stomatol. Oral Maxillofac. Surg.* **2018**, *119*, 389–394. [CrossRef]
18. Nadella, K.R.; Kodali, R.M.; Guttikonda, L.K.; Jonnalagadda, A. Osteoradionecrosis of the Jaws: Clinico-Therapeutic Management: A Literature Review and Update. *J. Maxillofac. Oral Surg.* **2015**, *14*, 891–901. [CrossRef]
19. Studer, G.; Bredell, M.; Studer, S.; Huber, G.; Glanzmann, C. Risikoprofil für Osteoradionekrosen des Kiefers in der IMRT-Ära. *Strahlenther. Onkol.* **2016**, *192*, 32–39. [CrossRef]
20. Ben-David, M.A.; Diamante, M.; Radawski, J.D.; Vineberg, K.A.; Stroup, C.; Murdoch-Kinch, C.-A.; Zwetchkenbaum, S.R.; Eisbruch, A. Lack of Osteoradionecrosis of the Mandible After Intensity-Modulated Radiotherapy for Head and Neck Cancer: Likely Contributions of Both Dental Care and Improved Dose Distributions. *Int. J. Radiat. Oncol.* **2007**, *68*, 396–402. [CrossRef]

21. Anderson Head and Neck Cancer Symptom Working Group. Dose-volume correlates of mandibular osteoradionecrosis in Oropharynx cancer patients receiv-ing intensity-modulated radiotherapy: Results from a case-matched comparison. *Radiother. Oncol.* **2017**, *124*, 232–239. [CrossRef] [PubMed]
22. Dore, F.; Filippi, L.; Biasotto, M.; Chiandussi, S.; Cavalli, F.; di Lenarda, R. Bone scintigraphy and SPECT/CT of bisphos-phonate-induced osteonecrosis of the jaw. *J. Nucl. Med.* **2009**, *50*, 30–35. [CrossRef] [PubMed]
23. Mohamed, A.S.; He, R.; Ding, Y.; Wang, J.; Fahim, J.; Elgohari, B.; Elhalawani, H.; Kim, A.D.; Ahmed, H.; Garcia, J.A.; et al. Quantitative Dynamic Contrast-Enhanced MRI Identifies Radiation-Induced Vascular Damage in Patients With Advanced Osteoradionecrosis: Results of a Prospective Study. *Int. J. Radiat. Oncol.* **2020**, *108*, 1319–1328. [CrossRef] [PubMed]
24. Zaghi, S.; Miller, M.; Blackwell, K.; Palla, B.; Lai, C.; Nabili, V. Analysis of surgical margins in cases of mandibular oste-oradionecrosis that progress despite extensive mandible resection and free tissue transfer. *Am. J. Otolaryngol.* **2012**, *33*, 576–580. [CrossRef] [PubMed]
25. Alam, D.S.; Nuara, M.; Christian, J. Analysis of Outcomes of Vascularized Flap Reconstruction in Patients with Advanced Mandibular Osteoradionecrosis. *Otolaryngol. Neck Surg.* **2009**, *141*, 196–201. [CrossRef]
26. Curi, M.M.; dos Santos, M.O.; Feher, O.; Faria, J.C.M.; Rodrigues, M.L.; Kowalski, L.P. Management of Extensive Osteoradionecro-sis of the Mandible With Radical Resection and Immediate Microvascular Reconstruction. *J. Oral Maxillofac. Surg.* **2007**, *65*, 434–438. [CrossRef]
27. Marx, R.E. A new concept in the treatment of osteoradionecrosis. *J. Oral Maxillofac. Surg.* **1983**, *41*, 351–357. [CrossRef]
28. Kraeima, J.; Steenbakkers, R.J.H.M.; Spijkervet, F.K.L.; Roodenburg, J.L.N.; Witjes, M.J.H. Secondary surgical man-agement of osteoradionecrosis using three-dimensional isodose curve visualization: A report of three cases. *Int. J. Oral Maxillofac. Surg.* **2018**, *47*, 214–219. [CrossRef]
29. Kraeima, J.; Schepers, R.H.; van Ooijen, P.M.A.; Steenbakkers, R.J.H.M.; Roodenburg, J.L.N.; Witjes, M.J.H. Integration of oncologic margins in three-dimensional virtual planning for head and neck surgery, including a validation of the software pathway. *J. Cranio Maxillofac. Surg.* **2015**, *43*, 1374–1379. [CrossRef]

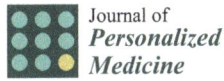

Journal of
Personalized
Medicine

Article

Three-Dimensional Guided Zygomatic Implant Placement after Maxillectomy

Nathalie Vosselman *, Haye H. Glas, Bram J. Merema, Joep Kraeima, Harry Reintsema, Gerry M. Raghoebar, Max J. H. Witjes and Sebastiaan A. H. J. de Visscher

Department of Oral and Maxillofacial Surgery, University Medical Center Groningen, University of Groningen, Hanzeplein 1, P.O. Box 30.001, 9700 RB Groningen, The Netherlands; h.h.glas@umcg.nl (H.H.G.); b.j.merema@umcg.nl (B.J.M.); j.kraeima@umcg.nl (J.K.); h.reintsema@umcg.nl (H.R.); g.m.raghoebar@umcg.nl (G.M.R.); m.j.h.witjes@umcg.nl (M.J.H.W.); s.a.h.j.de.visscher@umcg.nl (S.A.H.J.d.V.)
* Correspondence: n.vosselman@umcg.nl

Abstract: Zygomatic implants are used in patients with maxillary defects to improve the retention and stability of obturator prostheses, thereby securing good oral function. Prosthetic-driven placement of zygomatic implants is even difficult for experienced surgeons, and with a free-hand approach, deviation from the preplanned implant positions is inevitable, thereby impeding immediate implant-retained obturation. A novel, digitalized workflow of surgical planning was used in 10 patients. Maxillectomy was performed with 3D-printed cutting, and drill guides were used for subsequent placement of zygomatic implants with immediate placement of implant-retained obturator prosthesis. The outcome parameters were the accuracy of implant positioning and the prosthetic fit of the obturator prosthesis in this one-stage procedure. Zygomatic implants ($n = 28$) were placed with good accuracy (mean deviation 1.73 ± 0.57 mm and $2.97 \pm 1.38°$ 3D angle deviation), and in all cases, the obturator prosthesis fitted as pre-operatively planned. The 3D accuracy of the abutment positions was 1.58 ± 1.66 mm. The accuracy of the abutment position in the occlusal plane was 2.21 ± 1.33 mm, with a height accuracy of 1.32 ± 1.57 mm. This feasibility study shows that the application of these novel designed 3D-printed surgical guides results in predictable zygomatic implant placement and provides the possibility of immediate prosthetic rehabilitation in head and neck oncology patients after maxillectomy.

Keywords: maxillectomy; guided surgery; zygomatic implants; digital; 3D; prosthetic rehabilitation; head and neck oncology; maxillary tumor; maxillary reconstruction; 3D VSP

1. Introduction

Several reconstructive techniques are available for patients with complex defects of the mid-face and maxilla following tumor resection. The size and extent of the maxillary defect, patient factors, and comorbidities are decisive factors for the choice of surgical, prosthodontic, or combined rehabilitation after a maxillectomy. In cases when tumor resection has caused a relatively small maxillary defect, primary closure or surgical reconstruction with a local soft tissue flaps alone can lead to excellent functional and aesthetic results. For larger maxillary defects, reconstruction with a vascularized flap or prosthetic rehabilitation with an obturator prosthesis can be used, the latter remaining an important treatment in many institutions [1]. However, conventional obturator prostheses can have their drawbacks, mainly caused by lack of retention of the prostheses. Placement of endosseous implants in the native bone of the maxilla allow for improvement of retention of the obturator prosthesis and thereby increase the success of prosthetic rehabilitation. While there is often not enough bone volume for reliable implant placement, zygomatic implants can be used to improve the retention of the obturator prosthesis [1–3].

The literature reports good zygomatic implant survival rates (78.6 to 100%) after placing maxillary resections [4]. Primary implant placement at the time of ablative surgery

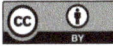

along with early loading of implants has been shown to be an effective rehabilitation protocol [1–3]. Although the survival rates are promising, this more complex treatment modality is not a standard implant procedure among many clinicians. Due to drilling with long drills close to critical anatomical structures, compromised visibility, and for oncological cases, also the absence of anatomical landmarks, the oblique drill trajectories for placement of zygomatic implants are challenging [5]. Inaccurate placement could result in uncontrolled bleeding, damage to the orbit and its content, damage to the maxillary sinus, and traumatic fractures to the orbitozygomatic complex [6,7]. Moreover, inaccurate placement and angulation of the implant results in positional errors at the apex and of the prosthetic head. This possibly results in an undesired prosthetic outcome and may even make the use of the zygomatic implant unattainable.

Pre-operative 3D planning and guided placement and drilling according to a virtual surgical plan could solve these problems and result in lower risk of complications compared to the free-hand approach. With the use of virtual implant planning, an optimal inclination, position, and depth of the zygomatic implant can be chosen considering volume and anatomical variation of the malar bone [8]. Moreover, the ideal prosthetic platform positions can be planned, which eliminates the possible need for the intraoperative "guess work" involved with complex zygomatic implant rehabilitation [9].

While there is widespread experience in guided placement of endosseous dental implants and guided resection of tumors, a proper tool for guided placement of zygomatic implants in maxillectomy patients is not yet available. With the combination of the oblique bone surface, the long drill trajectories and the extent of the defects make designing guided templates a challenge. Any small angular or positional entrance error results in magnification of apical positional error at the tip of the drill [10]. The drill guide for zygomatic implant placement, introduced by Vrielink et al. [11] in 2003, which was solely based on available bone volume, unfortunately had an unfavorable accuracy. A technical note describing guided placement of zygomatic implants in atrophic maxillae lacks implant placement-accuracy analysis [12].

Recently, our group described a novel design of a fully digital 3D surgical planning for accurately executing the ablative surgery, placement of zygomatic implants, and immediate placement of an implant-retained obturator prosthesis in human cadavers [13].Therefore, the aim of this study was to assess whether this full 3D virtual workflow to guiding zygomatic implants placement and providing the patient with a printed surgical obturator prosthesis in head and neck cancer patients with a maxillary defect would be clinically feasible.

2. Materials and Methods

A total of 10 consecutive patients (7 female, 3 male, mean age of 66.3 years, range 45–73 years) who were treated for oral malignancies at the department of Oral and Maxillofacial Surgery at the University Medical Center Groningen were included. Patients either had a pre-existing defect of the maxilla (n = 3) or were scheduled for a maxillectomy (n = 7) with reconstruction an obturator prosthesis supported by zygomatic implants. All maxillary defects in this study are categorized as a class Brown IIb defect [14]. Patient, tumor, and defect characteristics are described in Table 1. For all patients, a complete 3D virtual surgical planning was made, in which zygomatic implants as well as an implant-retained obturator prosthesis were included.

Table 1. Patient, tumor, and defect characteristics.

Patient	Age (Years)	Sex	Indication	Laterality	Implants	IMPL Length (mm)	Radiotherapy
1	49	F	cT4N0 Adenoid cystic carcinoma maxilla	R	2	42.5; 55	Post-op
2	73	F	cT1N0 Squamous cell carcinoma maxilla	R & L	4	52.5; 45; 52.5; 47.5	Pre-op Post-op
3	64	F	cT4aN1M0 Squamous cell carcinoma maxilla	R	4	55; 50	-

Table 1. *Cont.*

Patient	Age (Years)	Sex	Indication	Laterality	Implants	IMPL Length (mm)	Radiotherapy
4	74	M	pT4aN0M0 Melanoma cavum nasi	R	2	55; 55	Post-op
5	71	F	cT3N0M0 Oral lentiginous melanoma maxilla	R	4	35; 45; 42.5; 50	Post-op
6	67	M	T4N0 Squamous cell carcinoma maxilla	L	2	47.5; 55	Pre-op
7	60	F	cT4N0 Squamous cell carcinoma maxilla	R	2	47.5; 55	-
8	45	M	Langerhans Histiocytosis	R & L	4	55; 52.5; 55; 52.5	Pre-op
9	66	F	Osteosarcoma maxilla	R	2	45; 50	-
10	71	F	pT4aN0 Squamous cell carcinoma maxilla	R&L	4	55; 50; 55; 47.5	-

2.1. Pre-Implant Procedure and 3D Planning

Prior to ablative oncological surgery, each patient underwent a diagnostic work-up consisting of both a CT and MRI of the head and neck region for ablative surgery and implant planning. In dentate patients, the natural dentition of dentulous patients was digitalized through 3D optical surface scanning and could be matched to the 3D patient models. In edentulous cases, additional cone-beam-computed tomography scan (CBCT) datasets of the patients wearing their conventional prostheses were obtained. The patient's prosthesis was prepared before scanning: five radiopaque markers were added and spread over the prosthesis. Immediately after the scanning, a second scan of the prosthesis itself was performed. Through the radiopaque markers, the two CBCT-datasets of the patient and the prosthesis were merged to match the virtual prosthesis to the 3D models of the patient's anatomy.

By using a multi-modality CT and MRI combined workflow for 3D resection margin planning [15], the tumor was delineated on the MRI data, after which this dataset was fused with the CT bone data in order to construct a 3D bone and tumor model. This model enabled reliable virtual resection planning with oncologic margins [16]. The virtual patient dentition or prosthesis was matched to the virtual planning to allow for digital obturator prosthesis designing, matching the defect, and backwards planning of the zygomatic implants from the position of the obturator prosthesis. The zygomatic implant heads were placed in the most ideal prosthodontic positions. The apical part of the zygomatic implant was planned in the lateral cortical bone of the zygomatic complex with care for maximal bony contact of the implant. The needed length of zygomatic implant was determined. In dentate cases, two zygomatic implants were digitally planned at the maxillary defect site. Four zygomatic implants were planned in edentulous cases.

2.2. Guide Design

Translation of the 3D VSP towards the surgical procedure was realized by means of 3D-printed surgical guides (Figure 1).

Subsequently, patient-specific implant drill guides were designed based on the preferred apical and abutment positions of the zygomatic implants captured in the final virtual set-ups (3-Matic Medical, Materialise, Leuven, Belgium). In edentulous cases, the drill guides were developed to fit the alveolar ridge, nasal aperture, and zygomatic arch for stable positioning (Figure 2A,B).

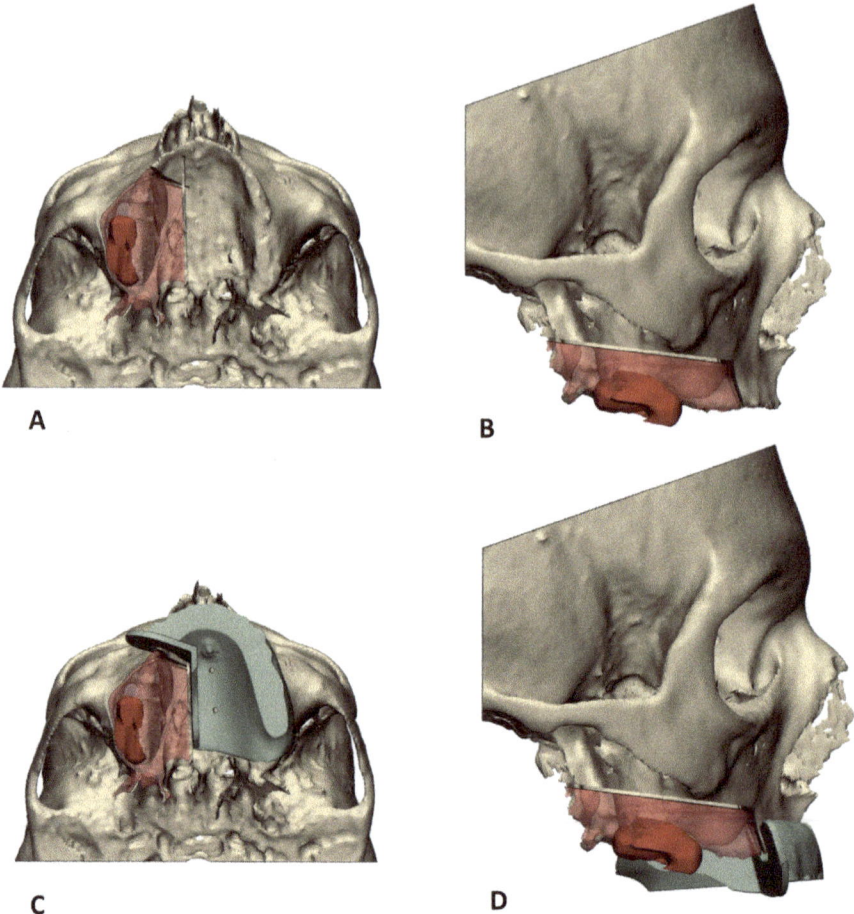

Figure 1. Overview of 3D VSP workflow for virtual resection planning. The working method starts with right-sided maxillectomy (**A**), caudal view (**B**), and the matching lateral view guided by the surgical cutting guides (**C,D**), with which the aim is to remove the red transparent part representing tumor removal with margin.

The maxillary bone-supported part included an extension to the nasal aperture to verify correct positioning of the guide [17] and was connected with crosslink arms to the zygomatic bone-supported part. Centered channels in the drill-guides enable insertion of stainless steel milled drill sleeves, which should minimize deviation of the drill trajectories and prevent polyamide particle formation (Figure 2C,D). The length of the channels functions as an integral depth stop for the zygomatic implants (Figure 2E,F).

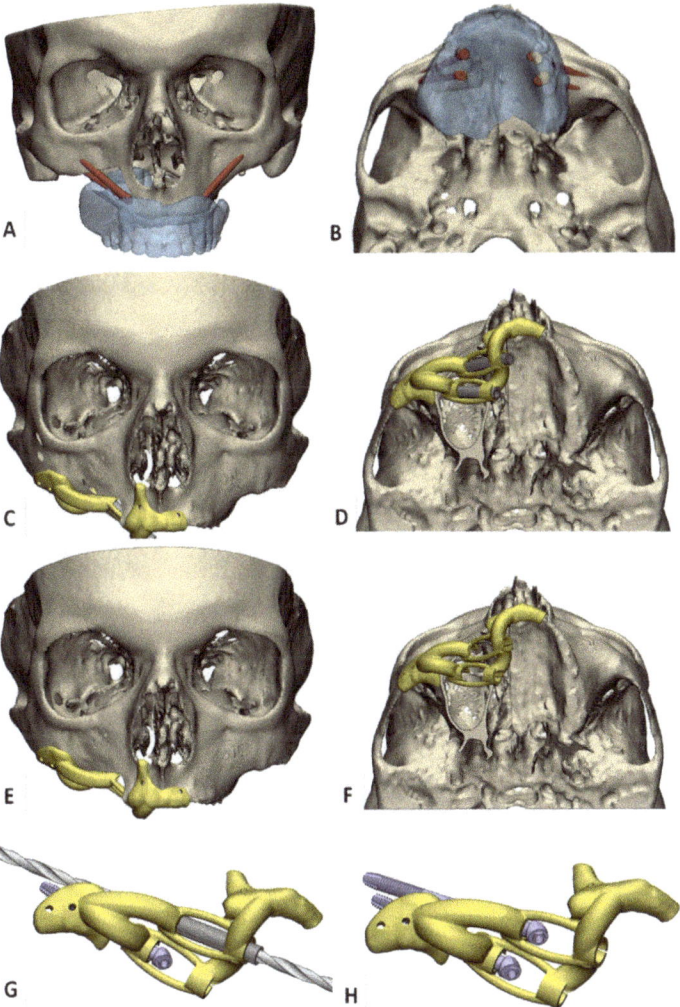

Figure 2. Overview of 3D VSP workflow for virtual zygomatic implant planning. (**A,B**) Virtual obturator prosthesis-driven zygomatic implant planning in an edentulous patient with right-sided maxillary resection planning. (**C,D**) Bone-supported zygomatic implant drill guide. Support is gained at alveolar ridge, nasal aperture, and zygomatic arch for stable positioning, and centered channels in the drill-guide enable insertion of stainless steel milled drill sleeves. (**E,F**) the length of the channels forms an integral depth stop for the zygomatic implants. (**G**) detailed view of drill guidance. (**H**) detailed view of zygomatic implants placed through the guide to enhance correct prosthetic head positions.

In addition, the guide was supplied with holes for temporary fixation with mini screws. If natural dentition was remaining after resection, the teeth were used for support of the guides (Figure 3). The guides were printed from polyamide, produced according to the ISO 13485 standards for medical devices, by Oceanz (Ede, The Netherlands).

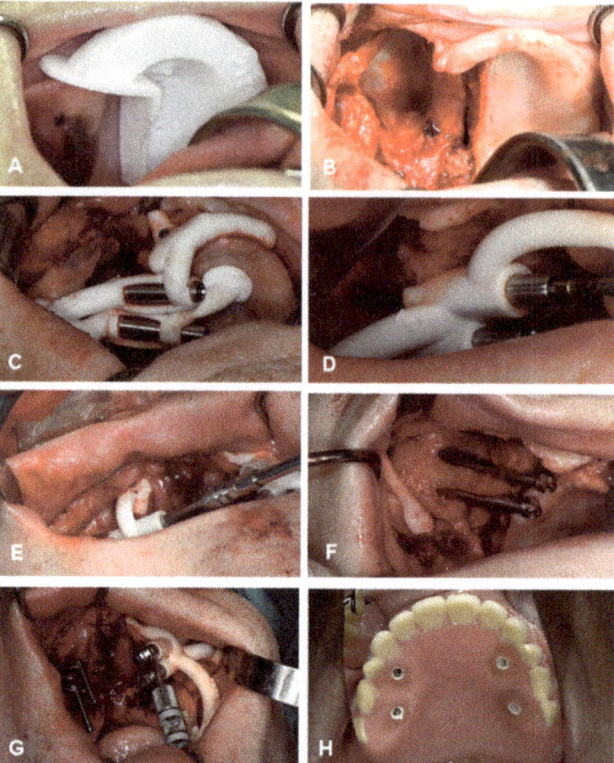

Figure 3. Surgical procedure. (**A**,**B**), maxillectomy according to the preplanned, individually designed cutting guides. (**C**) Drill guide seated with a tight fit and fixated with osteosynthesis screws. (**D**) Zygomatic drill inserted in the guide to perform the preplanned drill. (**E**) Insertion of zygomatic implant into the bone until the fixture mount contacts the reference stop on the guide. (**F**) View of zygomatic implant positions after removing the guide. (**G**) Final screw direction of the fixture mounts, which correspond exactly with the abutment positions. (**H**) Implant-retained obturator prosthesis immediately fixated with non-engaging prosthetic cylinders mounted into the prepared slots with a light-curing denture resin.

2.3. Surgical Procedure

First, the tumor was removed by resecting the maxilla (SV) according to the preplanned, individually designed cutting guides (Figure 3A,B). In the two cases in which the maxillectomy already had been performed, a mucoperiosteal flap was raised. Second, the zygomatic implant drill guide was fitted onto the bone. All zygomatic implants were placed by the same surgeons (S.V. and G.R.). During exposure of the maxillary and zygomatic bone, care was taken in order to remove all connective tissue from the guide supporting bone region so that the drill guide could be seated with a tight fit. The guide was fixated with osteosynthesis screws (KLS Martin, Tuttlingen, Germany) (Figure 3C). Third, the first metal sleeves matching the 2.7 mm zygomatic drill with apical lance were inserted in the guide to create the entry point in the malar bone. Subsequently, the preplanned drill trajectories were performed (Figure 3D). The metal sleeve was removed, which transformed the guide into a placing guide for the correct installation angle for the zygomatic implants (Zygex, Southern implants, Gauteng, South Africa). Next, the implants were inserted into the zygomatic bone until the fixture mounts contacted the reference stop on the guide. (Figure 3E). Due to longitudinal slots in the guide, the guide can be removed easily following implant placement by loosening the osteosynthesis screws and unclipping the guide from the implants (Figure 3F). Before removing the guide, the maxillofacial prosthodontist determines the final screw direction of the fixture mount, which corresponds exactly with the abutment position (Figure 3G). The obturator prosthesis with preplanned slots can be used as a reference to ensure a parallel positioning of the prosthetic platforms. In the edentulous cases ($n = 5$), a second guide was placed on the contralateral side, and the guided implant procedure was repeated. The surgical procedure was finalized by fixating the obturator prosthesis. Non-engaging prosthetic cylinders (Southern implants, Irene) were fixed to the obturator prosthesis with ultraviolet light-curing resin. The obturator prosthesis was checked for balance support and was firmly screw-fixed on the zygomatic implant abutments (Figure 3H). The screw-retained retention allows post-operative removal of the surgical obturator prosthesis and enables replacement as often as necessary

2.4. Analysis of Accuracy

All patients underwent a routine postoperative cone-beam-computed tomography scan (CBCT) within 16 days after surgery, which was used to evaluate the accuracy of the implant placement. The computer-aided design (CAD) files in STL format of the titanium zygomatic implants were superimposed onto the postoperative CT data, and a comparison was made with the planned positions by calculating reproducible reference planes in which the accuracy was measured. The implant coordinate system (ICoS) includes three reproducible reference planes in which the accuracy was measured: the center of the zygomatic implant head, bone entry point of the implant, and bone exit point of the implant (Figure 4A). Furthermore, the 3D angular deviation between 3D-planned position and postoperative implant position was calculated (Figure 4B).

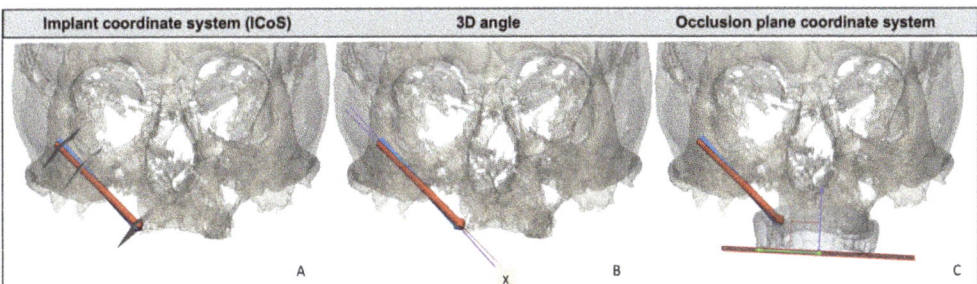

Figure 4. Overview of the different types of measurements and reference planes or coordinate systems for assessing the accuracy of zygomatic implant placement derived from post-op CBCT. In red, the planned zygomatic implant position; in blue, the postoperative zygomatic implant position. (**A**) The implant coordinate system (ICoS), including the three reproducible reference planes in which the accuracy is measured: the center of the zygomatic implant head, bone entry point of the implant, and bone exit point of the implant. (**B**) 3D angular deviation between 3D-planned position and postoperative implant position. X represents the 3D angle deviation. (**C**) Occlusion plane coordinate system. A plane parallel to the prosthetic occlusional plane is defined; perpendicular to this plane is the blue arrow. This arrow indicates the direction in which the abutment height accuracy is calculated. Deviation of the abutment is measured in the occlusional plane (green arrow).

Deviation of abutment position in two dimensions were calculated by defining a plane parallel to the prosthetic occlusional plane as reference: the occlusion plane coordinate system (Figure 4C). If the implant-retained obturator prosthesis on the zygomatic implant abutments was within 3 mm of the prosthetic cylinders in the slots, and a passive fit could be achieved, placement was deemed a success.

3. Results

3.1. Implant Placement Accuracy

The surgical guides fitted well in 9 cases (28 zygomatic implants). In one case, the fit of the surgical guide was not optimal because a larger resection of the tumor than planned was performed. These two implants were placed non-guided and therefore eliminated from the accuracy analysis. The implant lengths varied between 35 mm and 55 mm and were placed with a mean entry point deviation of 1.73 ± 0.57 mm and a 3D angle deviation of $2.97 \pm 1.38°$ (range 0.6–6.1°). The 3D accuracy of the abutment positions was 1.58 ± 1.66 mm. The accuracy of the abutment position in the occlusal plane was 2.21 ± 1.33 mm, with a height accuracy of 1.32 ± 1.57 mm. An overview of the accuracy results can be seen in Tables 2 and 3. The accuracy was well within tolerance limits.

Table 2. Accuracy data. Result of the post-operative analysis of the implant coordinate system (ICoS) measurements. * SD, standard deviation.

ICoS Measurements $n = 10$	Mean (+/− * SD)	Min	Max
Abutment (mm)	1.60 (+/−0.64)	0.53	3.42
Entry point (mm)	1.81 (+/−0.64)	0.43	3.24
Exit point (mm)	2.87 (+/−1.18)	1.11	4.72

Table 3. Accuracy data. Result of the post-operative analysis. Descriptive statistics of the occlusion coordinate system (OCoS) measurements. * SD, standard deviation.

OCoS Deviations $n = 10$	Mean (+/− * SD)	Min	Max
Abutment in occlusal plane (mm)	2.45 (+/−1.35)	0.87	6.04
Abutment height from occlusal plane (mm)	1.58 (+/−1.66)	0.01	6.58
Axial angle (°)	2.31 (+/−1.52)	0.19	4.34
Coronal angle (°)	2.43 (+/−1.73)	0.25	7.97
Sagittal angle (°)	2.85 (+/−1.88)	0.27	7.04
3D angle (°)	3.20 (+/−1.49)	0.34	6.13

3.2. Fit of the Implant Retained Obturator Prosthesis

In nine cases, the obturator prostheses could be fixated with non-engaging prosthetic cylinders (Zygex Southern implants, Gauteng, South Africa) to the zygomatic implants as planned. The prosthetic outcome in the horizontal and vertical dimension was within the 3 mm leeway space. This margin was available in prepared slots of the obturator prostheses needed for fixation. In the case where the zygomatic implants were not guided placed, extensive prosthetic adjustments at the preplanned slots were needed to allow for a proper fit of the obturator prosthesis.

Finally, all pre-operatively designed obturator prostheses had an adequate and were well-balanced on the zygomatic implants and remaining maxillary structures.

4. Discussion

This feasibility study shows that the application of 3D-printed surgical guides results are feasible in predictable zygomatic implant placement and immediate prosthetic rehabilitation in head and neck oncology patients after maxillectomy. Furthermore, application of this reliable method is believed to minimize the risk of surgical and prosthetic complications.

The literature reports loading of zygomatic implants within a few hours after implant placement [18,19], but to the best of our knowledge, such a CAD workflow involving immediate implant-retained prosthetic rehabilitation in a combined surgical procedure with guided tumor resection and placement of zygomatic implants is not described. Thereby, comparative accuracy data are not available yet. Perioperative prosthetic delivery obviates invasive impression taking in surgical field or shortly after surgery, which is a direct benefit for the patient.

In the literature, an unfavorable zygomatic implant position of the apex or prosthetic head is described as a surgical complication [2,7]. This could indicate that even when executed by experienced surgeons, there is a frequent occurrence of suboptimal zygomatic implant positioning using a free-hand placement. The concept of guided zygomatic implant placement was first tested by our group in a series of human cadavers [12]. The data of this pre-clinical cadaver study and the data presented here are comparable in accuracy. As a consequence, immediate implant support was available for the obturator prosthesis.

This phase I trial shows high clinical potential for this approach of 3D-planned placement of zygoma implants. We think that a larger group of patients is required to confirm our first data on the predictability of placement and subsequent immediate loading of the obturator prosthesis. The lessons learned from this trial are that 3D planning can be accurately used when surgeons and prosthodontists together plan the surgery and prosthetic rehabilitation. 3D visualization of the tumor and planned resection promotes clinical debate and facilitates choices. The execution of the resection is less of a determining factor. Added resections are very well possible since the support for the 3D zygoma guides are chosen outside the expected oncological surgical field. Two factors are critical for accurate placement of the zygomatic implants. The first is the accurate placement of the 3D guide. Surgeons should be aware how the guides should be placed and 3D information should be available in the OR. Time must be taken to place these correctly, as is the case with all 3D-planned surgical guides for another purposes. Second, during placement of the implants, the surgeon should have the possibility of visual inspection of the entry point in the zygoma. Despite accurate 3D planning and well-thought out guide design, the surgeon needs visual feedback on the entry point. Once the entry point is placed accurately, the rigid guide supports the right direction of the implant drill.

Besides guided placement of implants, currently, implant placement using real-time navigation is gaining popularity. Research results are promising, and this most likely accurate and less-invasive surgical technique could be a next step in zygomatic implant placement according to a VSP in the future. To date, the main drawback of current visualization techniques is the difficulty of steadily maintaining the drill handpiece and transferring the surgical view from the navigation display to the operative site, which is amplified in the long drills used for zygomatic implants [20]. Secondly, it currently involves above-average operating time [9].

It is reasonable to assume that knowledge of the planned resection automatically provides 3D visualization of the necessary obturator outline to restore oral function. In this study, a treatment protocol was used for immediate prosthetic rehabilitation with immediate loading of the zygomatic implants. Restoring oral function immediately after ablative surgery obviates the need for fitting, placing, and adapting the prostheses. After maxillectomy, the frequent necessity of adjuvant radiotherapy limits the possibility of achieving sufficient retention for a conventional obturator prosthesis. An implant-retained obturator prosthesis allows for repeated removal to check the oncological defect visually or in the event of complications. The addition of subsequently placing a fixed, removable obturator prosthesis during surgery is a major step to shortening the time of prosthetic delivery and implant utilization. It can be anticipated that the number of prosthetic interventions post-operatively will be less compared to conventional prosthetic planning, in which retention is more difficult to obtain. We anticipate that oral function in such patients can recover earlier and better before the often necessary radiotherapy starts, and the hospital visits for prosthetic aftercare will be minimized in the early post-operative phase. In case of adjuvant radiotherapy, it is important to provide zygomatic implant-specific information to the radiotherapy team. This enables adjustments of the radiotherapy treatment plan and the dosimetric accuracy in radiotherapy [21,22].

5. Conclusions

A fully digitalized workflow for guided resection, zygomatic implant placement, and immediate prosthetic rehabilitation is feasible when planning a zygomatic implant-retained prosthesis. The method presented here is novel and advantageous for head and neck cancer patients because of an immediate implant-based prosthetic rehabilitation after ablative surgery, which otherwise could not have been achieved without delay.

Author Contributions: Conceptualization, N.V., H.H.G. and S.A.H.J.d.V.; formal analysis, H.H.G.; investigation, N.V., H.R., G.M.R., M.J.H.W. and S.A.H.J.d.V.; software, H.H.G., B.J.M. and J.K.; validation, H.H.G.; visualization, B.J.M.; writing—original draft, N.V. and H.R.; writing—review and editing, J.K., G.M.R., M.J.H.W. and S.A.H.J.d.V. All authors have read and agreed to the published version of the manuscript.

Funding: This research received no external funding.

Institutional Review Board Statement: The study was conducted in accordance with the Declaration of Helsinki and approved by the Ethics Committee of UMCG (reference M21.282070, 21 September 2021).

Informed Consent Statement: Informed consent was obtained from all subjects involved in the study.

Data Availability Statement: The data presented in this study are available in Table 2. The raw data presented in this study are available on request from the corresponding author. Requests for materials should be addressed to N.V.

Conflicts of Interest: The authors declare no conflict of interest.

References

1. Vosselman, N.; Alberga, J.; Witjes, M.H.; Raghoebar, G.M.; Reintsema, H.; Vissink, A.; Korfage, A. Prosthodontic rehabilitation of head and neck cancer patients-Challenges and new developments. *Oral Dis.* **2021**, *27*, 64–72. [CrossRef]
2. Hackett, S.; El-Wazani, B.; Butterworth, C. Zygomatic implant-based rehabilitation for patients with maxillary and mid-facial oncology defects: A review. *Oral Dis.* **2021**, *27*, 27–41. [CrossRef]
3. Boyes-Varley, J.G.; Howes, D.G.; Davidge-Pitts, K.D.; Brånemark, I.; McAlpine, J.A. A protocol for maxillary reconstruction following oncology resection using zygomatic implants. *Int. J. Prosthodont.* **2007**, *20*, 521–531. [PubMed]
4. Butterworth, C.J. Primary vs secondary zygomatic implant placement in patients with head and neck cancer-A 10-year prospective study. *Head Neck* **2019**, *41*, 1687–1695. [CrossRef] [PubMed]
5. Ramezanzade, S.; Keyhan, S.O.; Tuminelli, F.J.; Fallahi, H.R.; Yousefi, P.; Lopez-Lopez, J. Dynamic-Assisted Navigational System in Zygomatic Implant Surgery: A Qualitative and Quantitative Systematic Review of Current Clinical and Cadaver Studies. *J. Oral Maxillofac. Surg.* **2021**, *79*, 799–812. [CrossRef] [PubMed]
6. Chrcanovic, B.R.; Albrektsson, T.; Wennerberg, A. Survival and Complications of Zygomatic Implants: An Updated Systematic Review. *J. Oral Maxillofac. Surg.* **2016**, *74*, 1949–1964. [CrossRef] [PubMed]
7. Aparicio, C.; López-Piriz, R.; Albrektsson, T. ORIS Criteria of Success for the Zygoma-Related Rehabilitation: The (Revisited) Zygoma Success Code. *Int. J. Oral Maxillofac. Implant.* **2020**, *35*, 366–378. [CrossRef] [PubMed]
8. Bertos Quílez, J.; Guijarro-Martínez, R.; Aboul-Hosn Centenero, S.; Hernández-Alfaro, F. Virtual quad zygoma implant placement using cone beam computed tomography: Sufficiency of malar bone volume, intraosseous implant length, and relationship to the sinus according to the degree of alveolar bone atrophy. *Int. J. Oral Maxillofac. Surg.* **2018**, *47*, 252–261. [CrossRef] [PubMed]
9. Ponnusamy, S.; Miloro, M. A Novel Prosthetically Driven Workflow Using Zygomatic Implants: The Restoratively Aimed Zygomatic Implant Routine. *J. Oral Maxillofac. Surg.* **2020**, *78*, 1518–1528. [CrossRef]
10. Wu, Y.; Wang, F.; Huang, W.; Fan, S. Real-Time Navigation in Zygomatic Implant Placement: Workflow. *Oral Maxillofac. Surg. Clin. N. Am.* **2019**, *31*, 357–367. [CrossRef]
11. Vrielinck, L.; Politis, C.; Schepers, S.; Pauwels, M.; Naert, I. Image-based planning and clinical validation of zygoma and pterygoid implant placement in patients with severe bone atrophy using customized drill guides. Preliminary results from a prospective clinical follow-up study. *Int. J. Oral Maxillofac. Surg.* **2003**, *32*, 7–14. [CrossRef] [PubMed]
12. Rigo, L.; Tollardo, J.; Giammarinaro, E.; Covani, U.; Caso, G. Fully Guided Zygomatic Implant Surgery. *J. Craniofac. Surg.* **2021**, *32*, 2867–2872. [CrossRef] [PubMed]
13. Vosselman, N.; Glas, H.H.; de Visscher, S.A.; Kraeima, J.; Merema, B.J.; Reintsema, H.; Raghoebar, G.M.; Witjes, M.J. Immediate implant-retained prosthetic obturation after maxillectomy based on zygomatic implant placement by 3D-guided surgery: A cadaver study. *Int. J. Implant Dent.* **2021**, *7*, 54. [CrossRef] [PubMed]
14. Brown, J.S.; Rogers, S.N.; McNally, D.N.; Boyle, M. A modified classification for the maxillectomy defect. *Head Neck* **2000**, *1*, 17–26. [CrossRef]

15. Kraeima, J.; Dorgelo, B.; Gulbitti, H.A.; Steenbakkers, R.J.; Schepman, K.P.; Roodenburg, J.L.; Spijkervet, F.K.; Schepers, R.H.; Witjes, M.J. Multi-modality 3D mandibular resection planning in head and neck cancer using CT and MRI data fusion: A clinical series. *Oral Oncol.* **2018**, *81*, 22–28. [CrossRef] [PubMed]
16. Kraeima, J.; Schepers, R.H.; van Ooijen, P.M. Integration of oncologic margins in three-dimensional virtual planning for head and neck surgery, including a validation of the software pathway. *J. Craniomaxillofac. Surg.* **2015**, *8*, 1374–1379. [CrossRef] [PubMed]
17. Onclin, P.; Kraeima, J.; Merema, B.J.; Meijer, H.J.; Vissink, A.; Raghoebar, G.M. Utilising the nasal aperture for template stabilisation for guided surgery in the atrophic maxilla. *Int. J. Implant Dent.* **2020**, *6*, 23. [CrossRef] [PubMed]
18. Maló, P.; Nobre Mde, A.; Lopes, A.; Ferro, A.; Moss, S. Five-year outcome of a retrospective cohort study on the rehabilitation of completely edentulous atrophic maxillae with immediately loaded zygomatic implants placed extra-maxillary. *Eur. J. Oral Implantol.* **2014**, *7*, 267–281. [PubMed]
19. Davó, R.; Malevez, C.; Rojas, J.; Rodríguez, J.; Regolf, J. Clinical outcome of 42 patients treated with 81 immediately loaded zygomatic implants: A 12- to 42-month retrospective study. *Eur. J. Oral Implantol.* **2008**, *9*, 141–150.
20. Wang, F.; Bornstein, M.M.; Hung, K.; Fan, S.; Chen, X.; Huang, W.; Wu, Y. Application of Real-Time Surgical Navigation for Zygomatic Implant Insertion in Patients With Severely Atrophic Maxilla. *J. Oral Maxillofac. Surg.* **2018**, *76*, 80–87. [CrossRef]
21. Puvanasunthararajah, S.; Fontanarosa, D.; Wille, M.L.; Camps, S.M. The application of metal artifact reduction methods on computed tomography scans for radiotherapy applications: A literature review. *J. Appl. Clin. Med. Phys.* **2021**, *6*, 198–223. [CrossRef] [PubMed]
22. Hansen, C.R.; Christiansen, R.L.; Lorenzen, E.L.; Bertelsen, A.S.; Asmussen, J.T.; Gyldenkerne, N.; Eriksen, J.G.; Johansen, J.; Brink, C. Contouring and dose calculation in head and neck cancer radiotherapy after reduction of metal artifacts in CT images. *Acta Oncol.* **2017**, *6*, 874–878. [CrossRef] [PubMed]

MDPI
St. Alban-Anlage 66
4052 Basel
Switzerland
Tel. +41 61 683 77 34
Fax +41 61 302 89 18
www.mdpi.com

Journal of Personalized Medicine Editorial Office
E-mail: jpm@mdpi.com
www.mdpi.com/journal/jpm

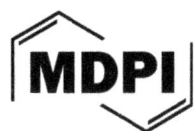

www.ingramcontent.com/pod-product-compliance
Lightning Source LLC
LaVergne TN
LVHW070613100526
838202LV00012B/642

9 7 8 3 0 3 6 5 6 4 8 4 5